New Directions in Irish and Irish American Literature

Series Editor
Kelly Matthews
Department of English
Framingham State University
Framingham, USA

New Directions in Irish and Irish American Literature promotes fresh scholarship that explores models of Irish and Irish American identity and examines issues that address and shape the contours of Irishness. The series aims to analyze literary works and investigate the fluid, shifting, and sometimes multivalent discipline of Irish Studies. Politics, the academy, gender, and Irish and Irish American culture have inspired and impacted recent scholarship centered on Irish and Irish American literature, which contributes to our twenty-first century understanding of Ireland, America, Irish Americans, and the creative, intellectual, and theoretical spaces between.

Holly May Walker-Dunseith

Traditional Medicine in the Irish Literary Revival

The Works of W.B. Yeats, Augusta Gregory, and J. M. Synge

palgrave
macmillan

Holly May Walker-Dunseith
University College Cork
Knock, Mayo, Ireland

ISSN 2731-3182 ISSN 2731-3190 (electronic)
New Directions in Irish and Irish American Literature
ISBN 978-3-031-82458-6 ISBN 978-3-031-82459-3 (eBook)
https://doi.org/10.1007/978-3-031-82459-3

This Palgrave Macmillan imprint is published by the registered company Springer Nature Switzerland AG.
The registered company address is: Gewerbestrasse 11, 6330 Cham, Switzerland

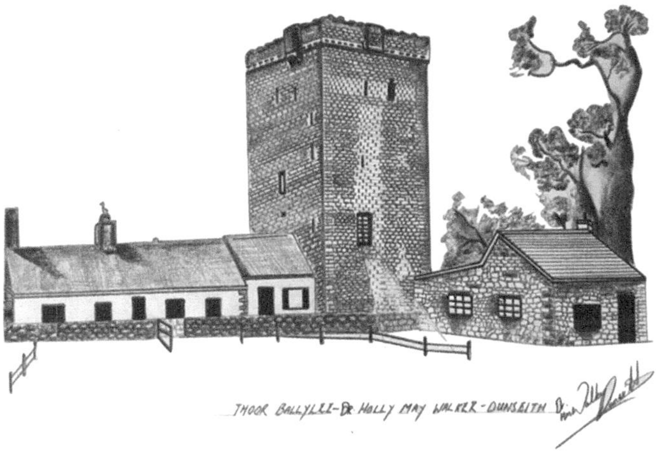

THOOR BALLYLEE – Dr. HOLLY MAY WALKER-DUNSEITH

Acknowledgements

This book is built on the support of the people that I here acknowledge. Firstly, thank you to my mum, Helen Dunseith, for her constant love and inspiration that she has given to me throughout my whole life. This book is dedicated to her. I also thank my dad, Colin Dunseith, for his love, support, and encouragement. I am grateful to my brother, Finn Walker Dunseith, for his kindness and humour. Thank you as well to a special schoolteacher, Mary Whitham, who laid the foundations of my education many years ago. Also, thank you to Sr Claire of Divine Mercy, the Carmelite Sisters, and Davina Morris for their friendship.

I would like to say a special thank you to my grandparents, Brian Walker and Kathleen Walker, who have been a big part of the journey of my life. I appreciate their love, support, and encouragement. Thank you to grandma Kathleen, uncle Harry Mitchell, and aunty Ann Mitchell for their information regarding natural Irish cures from my family.

I would like to thank my PhD supervisor, Dr. Adam Hanna, who gave me the opportunity to pursue the doctorate. I appreciate his expertise and advice. Thank you to Professor Alex Davis, who was also my PhD supervisor, for his expertise and advice.

I would like to thank University College Cork and especially UCC Library and the Special Collections and Archives department for providing me with research material. Thank you also to the *National Folklore Collection* at University College Dublin for their kind permission to reproduce quotations from their manuscript collections. Also, thank you to the John J. Burns Library at Boston College for providing the image of Yeats's annotations on AE's poem titled "The Well of All-Healing." I gratefully acknowledge the permission granted to reproduce the copyright material in this book. Every effort has been made to trace copyright holders and to obtain their permission for the use of copyrighted material. I apologise for any errors or omissions and would be grateful to be notified of them. Thank you also to Palgrave Macmillan in New York for publishing the book.

Thank you to Fr Richard Gibbons (Parish Priest and Rector of Knock Shrine) and Knock Museum at Knock Shrine for providing me with Venerable Archdeacon Cavanagh's *Diary of Cures* and collection of letters. Thank you very much to Fr Denis Hartnett for the interesting conversations and information about Christianity and the blessing of healing wells in Ireland.

Competing Interests The author has no competing interests to declare that are relevant to the content of this manuscript.

Praise for *Traditional Medicine in the Irish Literary Revival*

"Walker-Dunseith's study of Yeats, Gregory, and Synge constitutes a significant and original intervention in the growing body of critical literature on Irish Studies and medical humanities. Focusing on a representative range of their writing, she convincingly demonstrates the importance to her chosen authors of the practice of traditional folk medicine in their creation of literary works geared towards national revival and cultural rejuvenation."

Alex Davis, *University College Cork*

Contents

1 Introduction 1

Part I W. B. Yeats: The Search for the Land of the Young 15

2 A Wandering Path to Recovery: *The Wanderings of Oisin* (1889) 17

3 Thoor Ballylee: Healing and Recovery 57

Part II Augusta Gregory: From Colonies to Cough Medicines 89

4 Rejuvenation, Medicine, and Revival in the Works of Augusta Gregory 91

5 The Language of Healing Herbs 127

Part III J. M. Synge: Wells, Wellness and Well-Being 157

6 Synge and Congestion: The Respiratory System of the West 159

7 Healing Wells in the Work of John Millington Synge 175

8 Conclusion 193

Bibliography 199

Index 217

About the Author

Holly May Walker-Dunseith is an Irish author and researcher, who holds a PhD in Irish Literature and Medical Humanities from University College Cork in Ireland. She specialises in Irish literature, medical humanities, and theology. Her research includes a focus on the Irish Revival and representations of traditional medicine and healing practices in the work of W. B. Yeats, Augusta Gregory, and J. M. Synge. She holds a Master's Degree in Gaelic Literature (MA), also from University College Cork, as well as a Master's Degree in Theology (MTh) from St. Patrick's Pontifical University in Maynooth and the Carmelite Institute of Britain and Ireland in Dublin. She has worked as a fully qualified teacher of English at secondary level. Her teaching qualifications consist of a PGCE (Postgraduate Certificate in Education) with QTS (Qualified Teacher Status). Prior to her teaching career, she was awarded a BA (Hons) in English Language and Literature from the University of Leeds. She illustrates her own work and has published books, narrative, poetry, illustrations, and academic journal articles. She is the author of the illustrated book *Traditional Medicine in the Irish Literary Revival: The Works of W. B. Yeats, Augusta Gregory, and J. M. Synge* (2025). Her academic journal publications include "Revivalist: Medical Herbs and Rejuvenation in the Works of Lady Augusta Gregory" (2023) in *Estudios Irlandeses* and "The healer in the tower: Biddy Early and discourses of healing in the work of W. B. Yeats and Augusta Gregory" (2022) in the *Irish Studies Review*. Furthermore, her languages include Irish.

Abbreviations

CL 1	Yeats, William Butler. *The Collected Letters of W. B. Yeats, 1865–1895.* Edited by John Kelly and Eric Domville. Vol. 1, Clarendon P, 1986
CL 3	Yeats, William Butler. *The Collected Letters of W. B. Yeats, 1901–1904.* Edited by John Kelly and Ronald Schuchard, 1994. Vol. 3, Clarendon P, 1994
CW 8	Yeats, William Butler. *The Irish Dramatic Movement.* Edited by Mary FitzGerald and Richard J. Finneran, Scribner, 2003. Vol. 8 of *The Collected Works of W. B. Yeats*
CW 2	Synge, John Millington. *Prose.* Edited by Alan Price, Colin Smythe/Catholic U of America P, 1982. Vol. 2 of *J. M. Synge: Collected Works*
CW 3	Synge, John Millington. *Plays: Book I.* Edited by Ann Saddlemyer, Colin Smythe/Catholic U of America P, 1968. Vol. 3 of *J. M. Synge: Collected Works*
CW 4	Synge, John Millington. *Plays: Book II.* Edited by Ann Saddlemyer, Oxford UP, 1968. Vol. 4 of *J. M. Synge: Collected Works*
DIB	*Dictionary of Irish Biography*, Royal Irish Academy
NFC	*National Folklore Collection, The Main Manuscript Collection*, University College Dublin
NFCS	*The Schools' Manuscript Collection*, University College Dublin
NLI	National Library of Ireland, Dublin
NYPL	New York Public Library, New York
OED	*Oxford English Dictionary*, Online
VPl	*The Variorum Edition of the Plays of W. B. Yeats.* Edited by Russell K. Alspach, assisted by Catharine C. Alspach, Macmillan, 1966
VP	*The Variorum Edition of the Poems of W. B. Yeats.* Edited by Peter Allt and Russell K. Alspach, Macmillan, 1957
YL	Yeats Library Collection, National Library of Ireland, Dublin

CHAPTER 1

Introduction

This study is an investigation of the representations of traditional medicine in Revival-era literature, with a particular focus on the works of William Butler Yeats (1865–1939), Lady Augusta Gregory (1852–1932), and John Millington Synge (1871–1909). Folk medicine and cures, both image and metaphor, are central to the literature of what has become known as the Revival period in Ireland (c. 1889–1922).[1] This is an element of these writers' concerns with folk practices, and yet the Irish Literary Revival can be seen as a resuscitation of sorts: a cultural process that was framed in explicitly medical terms, which sought to breathe new life into the country's past. As John Wilson Foster wrote, "Recovery of the legends was recovery of a heroic Ireland, and recovery not merely in the sense of unearthing but in the sense of vigorous convalescence, of enabling a rebirth" (*Fictions* 10). Traditional medicine was a distinctive area of Irish life and practice that could be woven into Irish prose, drama, and poetry as part of the project of bringing to light the country's overlooked folk ways. The deployment of folk medicine, healers, and cures as an image,

[1] I discuss the periodisation of the Revival in Chapter Two, with reference to Norreys J. O'Conor's article "Ireland's Literary Revival and Regional Writing" (1947), Declan Kiberd and P. J. Mathews's book *The Handbook of the Irish Revival* (2015), and Laura O'Connor's chapter "W. B. Yeats and Modernist Poetry" in *The Cambridge Companion to Irish Modernism* (2014).

H. M. Walker-Dunseith, *Traditional Medicine in the Irish Literary Revival*, New Directions in Irish and Irish American Literature,
https://doi.org/10.1007/978-3-031-82459-3_1

though, had a metaphorical significance that is inextricable from the wider political tensions at work in Ireland in the decades before the foundation of the Free State. Literature that represents traditional medicine at times gestures towards the possibility of a culture and nation in the act of healing itself from illness, and at times questions these nationalist discourses.

This book is a contribution to the field of medical humanities in Ireland and, as such, is in conversation with existing medical humanities literature. From its outset, this sub-discipline has been concerned with the scientific or clinical setting. Michel Foucault's *The Birth of the Clinic: An Archaeology of Medical Perception* (1963) is, in Foucault's own words, "about space, about language, and about death; it is about the act of seeing, the gaze" (ix). This gaze falls in the attempted antiseptic conditions of the clinic, and it is therefore a very different study from one concerned with the spaces and contexts in which folk medicine was traditionally practised. Another key medical humanities text, Susan Sontag's *Illness as Metaphor* (1978), does not explore "physical illness itself" but looks at "the uses of illness as a figure or metaphor" (3). This is more germane to the present study, as this book is strongly concerned with the metaphors that connect body and nation. Sontag argues that "illness is *not* a metaphor, and that the most truthful way of regarding illness—and the healthiest way of being ill—is one most purified of, most resistant to, metaphoric thinking" (3). She goes on to state that "[i]t is toward an elucidation of those metaphors, and a liberation from them, that I dedicate this inquiry" (3–4). The present study is not concerned with liberation from metaphor so much as the uses to which medical metaphor is put. My research is contextualised within the field of medical humanities, but it extends the boundaries of this discipline by looking at the Irish Revival, a literary movement in which traditional medicine was of central importance.

Irish medical humanities literature is an apt context in which to place my study. A key text in this field is *The Body in Pain in Irish Literature and Culture* (2016), edited by Fionnuala Dillane, Naomi McAreavey, and Emilie Pine. This book, in the words of its editors, "elucidates the ways the pained and suffering body has been registered and mobilised in specifically Irish contexts across more than 400 years of literature and culture" (1). This specifically Irish context, I argue, must include a serious approach to folk medicine, including folk medical texts, the status of the healer, and the uses of healing plants. Using a plethora of sources (such as medical journals, folklore collections, letters, diaries, poems, plays, and prose), this study reveals new contexts and materials that both medical humanities and Revivalist scholars can employ.

Traditional medicine in Ireland in the nineteenth century was associated by writers with traditional Irish life, rural landscapes, countryside resources, and Irish identity. As such, it touched on some of the most treasured precepts of the Revival period. As the main precursor of writing in this field, Lady Jane Wilde's *Ancient Cures, Charms, and Usages of Ireland* (1890) was a key text on traditional medicine that later writers used to colour their literature with folk medical knowledge. This book is an enchiridion of traditional remedies that is something between a medical manual and a work of folk anthropology. The main claim that the book makes for itself, in Wilde's words, is that "the myths, superstitions, and legends (which are the expression of a people's faith), remain fixed and fast through successive generations, and finally become so inwoven with the daily life of the people that they form part of the national character and cannot be dissevered from it" (3). In the first half of the book, Wilde includes a detailed list that records traditional cures for specific medical conditions, which appears to form the central point of the work. However, Wilde then goes on to write down fictional peasant tales that weave medicine into myth. Wilde rejects the modern dichotomy between fictitious storytelling and what was believed at the time to be objective scientific information. Wilde combines the opposing concepts and marries traditional medicine and the *seanchaí* (storytelling) tradition. Through this method, Wilde laid the groundwork for other writers to build upon. Yeats often borrows from this source for his work, such as when he writes of hellebore and vervain in *The Countess Cathleen* (1892).

Lady Jane Wilde's works appear in both Yeats's and Gregory's libraries. Yeats owned her *Ancient Cures, Charms, and Usages of Ireland* (1890) and Edward O'Shea, the author of *A Descriptive Catalog of W. B. Yeats' Library* (1985), adds that the book is "[m]arked by WBY [William Butler Yeats]" with "[m]arginal markings, heavy, passim" (303). O'Shea records that there are "[m]any check marks against proverbs at the end of the book" (304). Yeats also owned both volumes of Wilde's *Ancient Legends, Mystic Charms, and Superstitions of Ireland* (1887) and, in the second volume, there are "[a] few annotations, not WBY's" (304). The importance of plants and herbalism to Augusta Gregory is shown by the fact that in her autobiography titled *Coole* (1971 [1931]), Gregory writes that "I sometimes ponder which among the volumes should I choose from their long accustomed places to go with me for the scanty years or days of eyesight and understanding that may remain" and John Evelyn's *Silva* (1786) is amongst these book choices (17; 20). This is important because Evelyn's book contained traditional herbal remedies, one of which was the forester's panacea, a medicine that he made for his neighbours. As I discuss in my chapter on Gregory, I find it likely that Gregory too made this remedy for the people who lived around her, based on the evidence that she made medicines for her neighbours, she treasured the book, and the herbal ingredients Evelyn writes of were readily available in her garden.

Writerly interest in traditional medicine was entwined with nationalism. Interest in it was a signifier of a political standpoint. In the nineteenth century, there was a widespread understanding of Irish heritage as sick and ailing, as can be seen from the many bodily metaphors that writers employed. Douglas Hyde, the President of Ireland from 1938 to 1945, includes metaphors of bodily decay in his famous speech "The Necessity for De-Anglicising Ireland" (1892):

> But in order to keep the Irish language alive where it is still spoken—which is the utmost we can at present aspire to—nothing less than a house-to-house visitation and exhortation of the people themselves will do; something, though with a very different purpose, analogous to the procedure that [Irish novelist] James Stephens adopted throughout Ireland when he found her like a corpse on the dissecting table. (qtd. in Kiberd and Mathews 44)

The use of metaphors of illness and death in descriptions of the body politic is perhaps not surprising. In *The Handbook of the Irish Revival: An Anthology of Irish Cultural and Political Writings, 1891–1922* (2015), Declan Kiberd and P. J. Mathews focus on the "deep paralysis" in "Irish life" and how "much of the impetus for this new movement for revival came from a heightened resolve to transcend the forces of decline and degeneration that had taken hold in Ireland throughout the nineteenth century" (32, 31).

This is reminiscent of James Joyce and his literary connection to paralysis, one of the central themes of *Dubliners*, most famously revealed when the unnamed boy in "The Sisters" reflects on Father Flynn's death and narrates in the first-person perspective: "I said softly to myself the word paralysis" (1). The persistence of these metaphors was perhaps related to the fact that public health in Ireland deteriorated after the Irish Famine (1845–1852). Starvation was the primary cause of a myriad of secondary diseases that plagued Ireland long after 1852. Chris Gilleard writes that "[f]ollowing the Great Famine of 1845–1849, it is argued, Ireland was transformed from a young, growing country to one that, by the end of the 19th century, had become 'prematurely' old" and that "Ireland experienced a premature 'ageing' of its society, with not only proportionately more people aged over 60 but also increasing sickness and a declining life expectancy amongst the over-60s" ("Other Victorians" 1157, 1158). During the Famine, Ireland was victim to a plethora of illnesses that emanated from hunger and poor living conditions, such as starvation dysentery, famine fever, cholera, and pneumonia.[2] Laurence Greary writes that "Famine-related deaths and emigration depleted the reservoir of disease in Ireland and the incidence of fever and other infectious diseases was significantly reduced in the wake of the disaster" ("Epidemic Diseases"). However, food shortages and the effects of poor diet and nutrition continued to surface. The Famine and the Penal Laws left behind long-lasting physical and emotional wounds that were deeply ingrained in the fabric of Ireland.

The post-Famine public health crisis in Ireland, specifically nutrition and living conditions, became a widespread public health topic. In *Reforming Food in Post-Famine Ireland: Medicine, Science and Improvement, 1845–1922* (2014), Ian Miller proposes that the time "between 1845 and 1880" was "a transformative period marked by public reflection on institutional living conditions" (66). He notes that "[p]hysicians paid closer attention to the issues of nutritional quality and deficiency and sought to firmly establish the potential long-term physical and mental consequences of consuming an insufficient diet" (65). The potato, vital for vitamin C and absorbing iron into the body, was "gradually replaced ... with less nutritious foodstuffs" (65). The New Poor Law (1838), enforced by the British government, was a moral depletion that

[2] Laurence Greary writes about illnesses that manifested during the Famine in his articles "Epidemic Diseases of the Great Famine" (1996) and "Deadly disease: how the Great Famine led to outbreaks of illness" (2020). The latter article is centred on John Crowley, William J. Smyth, and Mike Murphy's *Atlas of the Great Irish Famine* (2012). In both of his articles, Greary identifies the illnesses that were present during the Famine, which included: respiratory infections, pneumonia, bronchitis, lung problems, influenza, kidney issues, tuberculosis (phthisis), cholera, Asiatic cholera (1848–1849), smallpox, ophthalmia, measles, cos dubh (black leg), scurvy, dropsy, hunger oedema, chronic/starvation dysentery, bacillary dysentery, famine fever (relapsing and typhus fever), pellagra (of which dementia is a symptom), and diarrhoea ("Epidemic Diseases"; "Deadly disease").

enforced a "stigmatisation of poverty" (68). Under this law, "workhouse life" was centred "around the premise that institutional living conditions needed to be considerably worse than those endured by the able-bodied poor living outside of the workhouse" (68). Irish society was suffering from nutritional deficiency; Ireland itself was significantly mismanaged by a distant British administration.

Patrick Logan is a medical doctor, who gathered a collection of Irish remedies. *Making the Cure: A Look at Irish Folk Medicine* (1972) is a useful source when comparing traditional and conventional treatments. He recognises that, before modern medicine, folk medics, often called wise men and women, were affordable options for healthcare and "[a]t a time when few drugs had any curative effect, it mattered little if they were prescribed by a qualified doctor or a 'wise woman'; the confidence which went with the treatment made all the difference" (1, 3).[3] Logan notes that these dynamics were not confined to the past. In more recent times, "[w]ith the development of aseptic surgery, chemotherapy and antibiotics, doctors were inclined to forget that they were dealing with people" (4). He reflects upon the premise that "[f]olk curers, not having these material advantages, have not forgotten that they are treating people and therefore they continue to practice successfully because they bring reassurance" (4). Whilst Logan appreciates the importance of conventional medicine, he is aware that qualities from folk healers—such as reassurance and a patient-centred approach—can be brought forward into modern medicine.[4]

Ronnie Moore and Stuart McClean, in their introduction to *Folk Healing and Health Care Practices in Britain and Ireland: Stethoscopes, Wands and Crystals* (2010), record the difficulty in classifying "folk healing" as "it is a contested field" (6). It is debateable as to "what constitutes folk healing or, the more ubiquitous phrase in the literature, folk medicine" (6). In their study, they prefer to use the term "folk healing"

[3] Furthermore, in the article "Medical Writing in Irish," Aoibheann Nic Dhonnchadha highlights the significance of preventative care, and the high status and hereditary nature of Irish doctors, who were employed to serve affluent patrons (217, 219). She writes, "Professional medicine in the Gaelic world of the time was the preserve of a number of learned families who exercised their occupation on a hereditary basis" (217).

[4] Sinéad Garrigan Mattar is interested in primitivism and science. Her book *Primitivism, Science, and the Irish Revival* (2004) "look[s] in detail at the work of the first three directors of the Abbey Theatre—Yeats, Lady Gregory, and Synge—and in each case suggest[s] the nature of their personal primitivism and the extent to which it was influenced by comparative science" (2).

and aim to evoke "connotations less of the interventionist and curing aspects of the medical model, and more of the supplementary, caring aspects of the lay model" (6). In my study, I use "folk healing" and its associated semantic fields as descriptions of holistic care that encompasses both curing and caring as medical prisms.

In the chapter, "Folk Healing and a Post-scientific World," Moore and McClean propose that "[i]ndigenous medicine and folk healing extend back to prehistory and yet are practised throughout the modern world to a greater or lesser degree" (22). Tony Farmar, in his *Patients, Potions and Physicians: A Social History of Medicine in Ireland* (2004), explores the Royal College of Physicians of Ireland and its establishment in 1654. He argues that "from the earliest days of the College there was always a richly diverse medical marketplace, in which the patient was the initiator and buyer" (1). Far from a mainstream health care design, medicine was once a choice rather than a set system. In his article, "Believers, Sceptics, and Charlatans: Evidential Rhetoric, the Fairies, and Fairy Healers in Irish Oral Narrative and Belief" (2005), Timothy Corrigan Correll "examines storytelling events as contexts in which propositions about the fairies and folk healers associated with them were appraised and contested" and assesses that "traditions of belief and traditions of disbelief were competing discourses that came into collision" (1). Correll confirms that "[i]n nineteenth-century and early twentieth-century Ireland, magico-medical beliefs about the fairies and folk healers said to derive power from them were increasingly condemned on both rationalist and religious grounds" (1). Medical, folkloric, and literary texts provide a means of assessing the nature of Irish modernity at the outset of the twentieth century.

More recently, traditional Irish healing practices gained international prominence. Early in 2021, the *Genetic Engineering and Biotechnology News* published an article titled "New Antimicrobial Streptomyces Species Discovered in Irish Soil." This article reveals that Gerry A. Quinn has discovered a "soil used in ancient Irish folk medicine in the West Fermanagh scarplands" that "contains several species of antibiotic producing organisms." In response to the emerging issue of antibiotic resistance, the article reports that "[t]he urgent quest to discover new and chemically diverse antibiotics ... is therefore of topmost priority, and has led scientists to explore unconventional sources, including folk medicine." Each epoch revives folk medicine for its own purposes: whereas antibiotic resistance is a concern in our own age, ideas of nationalism and national revival were prevalent in the early twentieth century. The cures in the Irish countryside and terrain are by no means obsolete; they still hold a place in the modern world.

* * *

Ideas of health and revival are central to the works of Yeats, Gregory, and Synge; there are both personal and national concomitants in their work of all three. This book begins with the most celebrated writer in the Revival era, Yeats. The first section looks at images of traditional healing and the recovery of youth in his early work *The Wanderings of Oisin* (1889). "Wandering" is framed as both a legitimate medical symptom for memory disorders and is associated with a new mystical and spiritual epoch that rejects the predetermined courses of rationalism and materialism. Yeats presents wandering as a source of time-conquering strength, not illness or weakness, for his protagonist and Ireland. This word reveals Yeats's preoccupation with diminishment and old age, and it evidences the direct relationship between traditional folk medicine and the Irish Revival. The Irish countryside itself is represented as having a curative capacity. In this text, the western Irish countryside is yoked together with the medicinal herbs that are found there. The wheat, flowers, dandelions, and moss are curative; the herbs give a healing status to the entire countryside.

Yeats's incorporation of medicinal herbs into his work made their health-giving properties more visible. He gathered lore of traditional Irish medicine, a significant part of Ireland's rural history, and he applied it to a modern context in the hope that it would reconnect people to a sense of place and space that provides renewable medicine and an opportunity to heal from past wounds. Several years later, Yeats first wandered the area around Coole-Ballylee, collecting the broken fragments of Irish folklore and building them into a new indigenous body. Reclaiming wandering from a medical sign of weakness to a restorative quality of the spirit was an important part of Yeats's project. It was something that could be brought from the Land of the Young to a debilitated present-day Ireland. He was to find his real-life Tír na nÓg at Thoor Ballylee.

This section on Yeats, therefore, also investigates the restoration of Thoor Ballylee as a restoration back to health. In restoring this tower, he was tending to the primary aim of the Irish Literary Revival: to resuscitate and revive to full health an ailing Irish heritage. Through healing Thoor Ballylee, by extension, he was repairing a fractured Ireland following the Easter Rising (1916) and a wounded world following the First World War

(1914–1918). Not only is the tower somewhere that Yeats restored, but it is also a place that could, in his imagination, contribute to wider spiritual and societal restoration. Ideas of healing, revival, and recovery were built into the restored walls of Thoor Ballylee itself. Yeats's tower is a place of healing and renewal on a personal and national level. The landscape from which Thoor Ballylee rose had long been associated by Yeats with recovered health. In both 1896 and 1897, Yeats recovered from ill health whilst at Coole Park, which stood nearby. Yeats's first visit to the environs of Thoor Ballylee was in August 1896, and from his first encounter with the place it is associated with a narrative of recovery from ill health.

It is perhaps significant that Yeats recalled how Gregory sought to restore his strength through bringing him on folklore-collecting forays, as this practice itself sought to revive the subdued Irish energies that, in her eyes and those of other Revival-era writers, were falling prey to the encroachments of modernity. The thatched cottage that adjoins the stone tower connects it to the vernacular architecture of the locality, and that of the wider Irish countryside. Furthermore, the millboards that Yeats used in the tower's restoration link the building to a local myth of healing, and to the practitioner Biddy Early (1798–1874). Accounts of folk healers, like Biddy Early in Yeats's *The Celtic Twilight* (1893), connect this herbal practitioner to the healing moss that was reported to grow at an intersection of the millwheels at Yeats's Thoor Ballylee (*Mythologies* 14). Both physically and symbolically, Early is embodied in the building itself through the construction materials, the poetic voice, and the healing moss that weaves these ingredients together. Just as ligaments join bone to bone, Early is the connective tissue that links folklore and medicine. A practitioner in words rather than medicine, Yeats rebuilds Thoor Ballylee as an amalgamation of fractures that might, in being re-set, heal stronger.

The next section is on Augusta Gregory. It is an investigation on how she imitated models and guides that she took from her locality: one was the folk healer Biddy Early. Another was Cathleen Ni Houlihan herself, the protagonist from the eponymous single-act play about a *cailleach* (the Irish word for a hag but also a sovereignty goddess associated with the territory of Ireland) who transforms from old to young. In Gregory's act of self-redefinition, following the death of her husband in 1892, she selected new role models and guises for her life. With her collaborator W. B. Yeats she dramatised a spiritual self-portrait in the form of Cathleen Ni Houlihan, who walks away from the action, young again, at the end of the play of that name. Both Biddy Early and Cathleen Ni Houlihan are forms of healer and when she reinvented herself, the model of healing woman was one on which she drew. Her interest in health is best expressed by both volumes of her folklore collection, titled *Visions and Beliefs in the West of Ireland* (1920), and her other writings on traditional medicine such as her chapter "Herb-Healing" in *Poets and Dreamers: Studies and Translations from the Irish* (1903). In "Seers and Healers" in the first series of *Visions and Beliefs*, Gregory recalls a time when she brought Yeats to a healer around the Connemara area, Fagan, who confirmed that his "*uncertain eyesight*" was not the result of a fairy curse (1: 103, 108). There is a sure link between her field research in the Irish countryside and the traditional medicine that she writes into her plays and prose.

Gregory's self-reinvention—from landlord to arch-Revivalist—has been a matter of interest to scholars. However, intertwined with this change was Gregory's remodelling of herself as a contemporary Biddy Early. There is a strong possibility that Gregory's cough cure, mentioned vaguely in her letters, was the forester's panacea, a universal remedy that she was very likely to have come across in her reading and the materials for which she certainly held in her environs. Also, long before Yeats became her neighbour in 1917, when he bought Thoor Ballylee after negotiating its purchase throughout 1916, he exhibited medical complaints that rendered him dependent on Gregory's care. When Yeats and Gregory were writing, the elements of Irish legend and mythology that they focused on were the ones relating to ageing and death (and a fantasy of renewal). Theirs was in some ways a meta-Revivalist practice, reviving ancient stories about revival. Based on the rejuvenated *cailleach* and the folk healer, Gregory put into practice a new lifestyle that focussed on reviving Ireland, restoring the health of her neighbourhood, and challenging colonialism.

This section focuses on *The Pot of Broth* (1904). This is a Yeats-Gregory collaboration that showcases Gregory's knowledge that she learned from Bridget Ruane who was a local Irish herbalist and a key source for Gregory's "Herb-Healing" chapter in *Poets and Dreamers* and the "Herbs, Charms, and Wise Women" section in the second series of *Visions and Beliefs*. By reading this play alongside Gregory's other writings on herbs, and in the light of her association with the healer Bridget Ruane, we can understand the tramp's role in the play better, and the role of non-elite women like Ruane in the creation of the culture of the Revival. We can also better understand Yeats and Gregory's theatrical project. Many of the herbs that Gregory lists and describes in these folklore collections are repurposed as literary ingredients that she and Yeats mix into *The Pot of*

Broth, as well as other plays, where they create a symbolic language of healing herbs. There is a metanarrative running through Yeats's and Gregory's works and drama: they aim to cure and heal the world from damaging, shallow materialism and introduce a new era in which the heart is valued over the head. This is the mindset that led to them founding a national theatre in Dublin at the start of a new century. Though this is often thought about in primarily political terms, they also had a view to creating a new world. Both writers wanted a global salvation, an act of remaking and rejuvenating the world-mind.[5] This project of rejuvenation and recovery tied in with nationalistic beliefs, but also extended into the wider world too.

I argue that Gregory's reference to herbs becomes a language that is not only used as a form of communication in this collaborative play, but it also re-surfaces in another of her plays, *The Golden Apple: A Play for Kiltartan Children* (1916). Ireland was a wellspring for this transformative vision, but it was not its limit. The settings Yeats and Gregory employed were Irish; the language their protagonists spoke was distinctive to Ireland, yet the kind of recovery that Yeats and Gregory envisioned would have relevance far beyond the country's shores. Ruane was an accessible muse who gave Gregory the materials from which to craft a new language and set of preoccupations, and the tools with which to reshape herself as an inheritor and communicator of herbal knowledge. Ruane's service to Gregory was to teach her traditional medicine; Gregory preserved her medical memory in written format, without which, Ruane would most likely be lost in the shadow of Early. At the same time as she was learning of herbs from Ruane, these healing plants sprouted in her literary work. Gregory's knowledge that she learnt from Ruane's herbal expertise is traceable in *The Pot of Broth*. At the same time as Lady Gregory was innovating a new literary language based on her locality in the west of Ireland, she created a symbolic language of healing herbs. Gregory's folklore collections, specifically in relation to herbs, formed a foundation for her entire literary career and gave her a form of communication that could reach a universal audience. By writing *Poets and Dreamers* and *Visions and Beliefs* (this twenty-year gap constituted the next phase of a transformation that was, this time, strictly medical), Gregory induced a delayed popularity

[5] In his article titled "Yeats and Spirituality," Ronald Schuchard "think[s] of Yeats's life as a spiritual drama" (325).

for her herbalism teacher Ruane and brought her knowledge of healing and cures into the compass of the Irish Revival.

The final section of this book explores how John Millington Synge uses a *well* to explore his personal definition of *well*-being. Synge wrote plays, collected folklore, and had a keen interest in the environment around him. In *The Well of the Saints* (1905), he employs "well" as a homonym to mean both the literal well and to describe good health. This five-act play includes references to blindness and healing practices: a blind couple have the opportunity for their eyesight to be restored, but they reject this cure and choose to remain sightless. For Synge, the physical body of the well is a microcosm for the wider metaphysical concept of wellness. Synge was caught in the middle of contemporary well-being philosophies and ethics that looked at decision-making based on selfishness and happiness rather than virtue and intrinsic goodness. Whilst the well is a focal healing point for the community, Synge instead drew from the well of the self.

This book seeks to connect this play to contemporary developments. In 1891, the British government diagnosed congestion in rural Ireland and administered a treatment: they decided to establish the Congested Districts Board, which undertook action to alleviate hardship in remote areas and make the west of Ireland more economically sustainable. Synge criticised the Board as a colonised way of viewing the districts and a blind standardised modernity that had been imposed on the west of Ireland. The "Congested" part of the "Congested Districts Board" did not only apply to the remote areas of Ireland but it also had personal and metaphorical associations for Synge in a medical sense. Due to his asthma and experience of chronic illness, Synge would have been aware of the medical denotation of the word "congested" and he would have been all too familiar with its physical sensation of suffocation, a feeling that did not fit with the rural Irish districts that had never been congested in the first place and did not require the "cure" of decongestion (which was emigration). Synge employs "sight" as a concept that distinguishes eyesight from mindsight, objective from subjective perspectives, and confirms his view of well-being as separate from good physical health.

Holy wells, which are numerous in Ireland, are a useful lens with which to view medicine in Synge's works. Even though Synge's writing is ironic, he mentions places of healing in his play, such as Knock in County Mayo. It is likely that Synge knew about the healings at Knock that occurred in his lifetime, as they were well reported. John Millington Synge's first visit to the Well of the Four Beauties (Tobar an Ceathrar Álainn) on Inishmore

(Inis Mór), in 1898, is a place which was to become an inspiration for his play *The Well of the Saints* (1905). Healing wells are prevalent in Ireland and there are many accounts of people being cured using the water from these wells. The well that Synge encountered is renowned for healing blindness, a malady that would take on a central thematic role in his play *The Well of the Saints*.

Synge's fascination with healing wells, and the transformative possibilities that they represent, perhaps stems from his own ailments that he experienced from childhood. Synge, who had asthma, was familiar with illness; his health difficulties were subsequently woven into the fabric of his plays. However, he is not the only Revival-era writer who is interested in healing wells: Yeats, Gregory, and Wilde also draw from the rich history of wells as sources of healing in Irish life. Like Synge, Gregory experiments with the homonyms of "well" as both a source of healing water and a health state. Gregory, unlike Synge, treats the healing wells with a profound respect for both the saints associated with them as well as their important role in Irish life. To Synge, however, healing water from the west is an ambiguous substance, and its representation is a way of questioning both the Irish Revival and the homogenising capacities of modernity.

The abstract noun "revival" is "[t]he action of reviving something after decline or discontinuance" and the recovery of strength ("Revival"; *OED*). "Resuscitation," similarly, is a medical term that indicates a "[r]evival, renewal, or restoration" ("Resuscitation"; *OED*). Standish James O'Grady (1846–1928), a founding figure in the Revival, made an accurate prediction in his *Early Bardic Literature, Ireland* (1879). He writes, "When the study of the Irish literary records is revived, as it certainly will be revived, the old history of each of these raths and cromlechs will be brought again into the light, and one new interest of a beautiful and edifying nature attached to the landscape, and affecting wholly for good the minds of our people" (11). This concept is applicable to Yeats, Lady Gregory, and Synge. Through their writings on traditional healing practices, they draw traditional ideas into the modern world. These Revival-era writers all have an aversion to a future that is homogenous, capitalist, and utilitarian. All three writers whose work I look at in this book were, in their distinct ways, motivated by a vision of what Ireland, and the world, could be.

PART I

W. B. Yeats: The Search for the Land of the Young

CHAPTER 2

A Wandering Path to Recovery: *The Wanderings of Oisin* (1889)

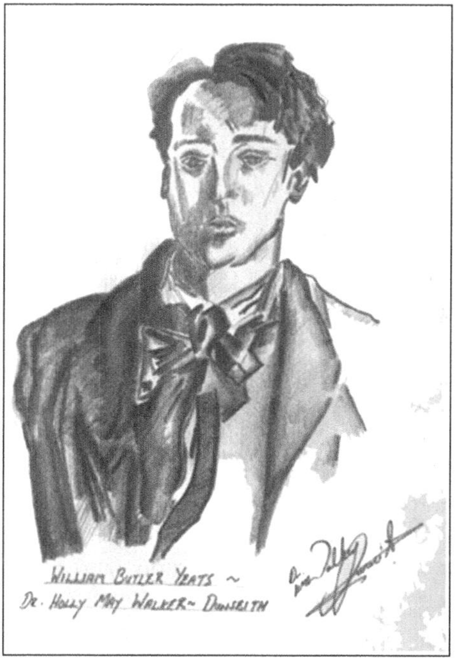

William Butler Yeats

H. M. Walker-Dunseith, *Traditional Medicine in the Irish Literary Revival*, New Directions in Irish and Irish American Literature,
https://doi.org/10.1007/978-3-031-82459-3_2

The titular character of *The Wanderings of Oisin* (1889) is an ambassador for a pagan, heroic past, who is feared and condemned by St. Patrick as he might embolden a country with his ancient memories. In many ways, this standard-bearer of an ancient tradition was a stand-in for Yeats who, like his fellow Revival-era writers, sought to bring the Promethean spark from Ireland's ancient past into its present day. Oisin, through his wanderings, has miraculously preserved his youth, and *The Wanderings of Oisin* bespeaks a wider project of restoring vigour and confidence to Irish culture. In this quest, Yeats presents wandering not as a symptom of illness or weakness, but as a source of strength.

Yeats's *The Wanderings of Oisin* is an epic poem, set in magical realms in Ireland, that focuses on a dialogue between St. Patrick and Oisin. It poses a contestation between worldviews. St. Patrick opens the poem by associating "wandering" with Oisin's bodily failure: he is, according to the saint, "bent, and bald, and blind, / With a heavy heart and a wandering mind" (*VP* book 1, lines 1–2).[1] Though the poem begins with the "wandering" being used in a deprecating sense, in his response to this, Oisin claims "wandering" back as a way of describing the eternal nature of story. To Oisin, stories are shifting, ghostly quantities that may at times fade but that perpetually revive their brilliance, like the moon. He diverts the conversation from bodily to literary wandering with the response "the tale, though words be lighter than air, / Must live to be old like the wandering moon" (book 1, lines 11–12). This initial response to Patrick reflects Yeats's role as a writer on the Celtic Twilight, a refresher and reviver of stories. Oisin reframes Patrick's perception of wandering as weakness and recasts it as a positive ethos—one that is flexible and free, unbound by the overly rational Victorian world. This positive meaning is reinforced shortly afterwards in a description of how the De Danaan, a legendary fairy race, "mock at Death and Time with glances / And wavering arms and wandering dances" (lines 274–75).[2] This wording is intriguingly close to the "[w]eaving olden dances, / Mingling hands and mingling glances" in Yeats's "The Stolen Child" (1889), which is a ballad with echoes of infant

[1] Unless otherwise declared, all poetry quotations for Yeats are taken from *The Variorum Edition of the Poems of W. B. Yeats* (1957), edited by Peter Allt and Russell K. Alspach.

[2] Mythologically, the Dé Danann race was believed to be an early set of fairy inhabitants of Ireland and were popularised as such in Irish literature. The Tuatha Dé Danann were "in Celtic mythology, a race inhabiting Ireland before the arrival of the Milesians (the ancestors of the modern Irish)" and "[t]he *Leabhar Gabhála* (*Book of Invasions*), a fictitious history of Ireland from the earliest times, treats them as actual people, and they were so regarded by native historians up to the 17th century" ("Tuatha Dé Danann"; *Encyclopædia Britannica*).

mortality (lines 17–18).[3] It is an early indication that Yeats presents wandering as a source of time-conquering strength, not illness or weakness, for himself and Ireland. Yeats and his fellow Revival-period writers were not just engaged in a nationalist project; it was one that sought to summon the energies of another epoch, another cast of mind and mode of thought and life. Key to it was "wandering"; it is something which could be a sign of weakness, but which Yeats seeks to redefine as a resistant Revival quality.

* * *

Wandering is central to Yeats's version of this ancient legend, set in prehistoric and pre-Christian Ireland. In it, both the eponymous Oisin and equally heroic Niamh travelled from Ireland to the Land of Youth, and thus became immortal whilst living in the undying environs. One hundred years later, Oisin finds a wooden staff from "some dead warrior's broken lance" and this reminds him of his Fenian comrades (book 1, line 367). Following analepses from his Irish past, Oisin and Niamh journey to the Island of Many Fears, and they battle a demon there for another one hundred years.[4] They spend a further century at the Island of Forgetfulness, where they fall into slumber and awake to sorrowful memories and "softness" that emanated "from the starlight" that fills Oisin "full to the bone" (book 3, line 72). When Oisin finally revisits Ireland, he discovers that the Fenians "ceased" in "old age" (line 177). Whilst en route back to the immortal lands, Oisin "fell on the path" and his "years three hundred fell" on him (lines 190, 191). St. Patrick then tells him he, like the other Fenians, is damned, whereupon Oisin defiantly tells him that he will "dwell in the house of the Fenians, be they in flames or at feast" (line 224). Oisin negotiates the boundaries between Heaven and Hell, past and present, and between wandering as a sign of weakness or wisdom.

* * *

[3] In the 1889 version of *The Wanderings of Oisin*, the line "And wavering arms and wandering dances" is absent from the text (*VP* line 275). It first appears in the revision of *The Wanderings of Oisin* in *Poems* (1895), where the new line reads as "And waving arms and wandering dances" (17). Therefore, the echo heard in "The Stolen Child" is in fact perhaps proleptic of Yeats's revision of *The Wanderings of Oisin/The Wanderings of Usheen* for the 1895 *Poems*. "The Stolen Child" may have prompted the revision to *The Wanderings of Oisin*. Yeats wrote the lyric during the composition of the first version of the longer poem.

[4] On departure from the Island of Many Fears, after deciding that their next destination was to be the Island of Forgetfulness, Oisin and Niamh mentioned other islands such as the "Islands of Dancing and of Victories" and the "Island of Content" (lines 247, 249).

Wandering is a state of mind, as well as a legitimate medical symptom for memory disorders, such as dementia, amnesia, and Alzheimer's disease. Medical wandering is a confused state whereby one wanders in speech, thought, and physically. For example: patients with Alzheimer's disease can physically wander due to fear of the environment, in search of the past, for basic needs, and in an effort to relive old routines (Dana Sparks and Mayo Clinic Staff). In other words, what looks to be wandering can in fact be a way of recovering a past state that is invisible to all but the wanderer. Patients with this condition are often prone to both mental and physical wanderings, where they remember an old memory and then attempt to travel to its geographical location. The aetiology of disorientation is memory disease, and this confusion can then culminate in wandering (Dana Sparks and Mayo Clinic Staff). These symptoms have a physiological cause in so far as they are products of the disease itself. Visio-spatial issues, for instance, mean that patients "can get lost even in familiar places because dementia affects the parts of the brain important for visual guidance and navigation" (Dana Sparks and Mayo Clinic Staff). "Wandering" is therefore associated medically with age and memory disorders, and it is viewed as a negative symptom in modern medicine.

Yeats, however, recruits the word "wandering" as a personal, metaphorical, and medical term that describes the process of remembering what has been forgotten and a mode of existence which the workaday contemporary world has forgotten to its cost. He reintroduces it into Irish society as an additional therapy in traditional medicine. From the outset, Patrick describes Oisin as having a "wandering mind," a symptom of illness on the brain (book 1, line 2). Oisin's wandering body, that is "bent, and bald, and blind," accompanies this fading mind (line 1). Even the hare "limps along in an aged whiteness," and the mouse "falters" as its "speed is a weariness" (lines 415, 421). Sickness and age continue as recognisable themes throughout the poem. The "kingfisher turns to a ball of dust, / And the roof falls in of his tunnelled house" and the "foam-white seagull drift[s] and float[s] / Under the roof, and with a straining throat" (book 1, lines 422–23; book 2, 105–06). If the "tunnelled house" symbolises a body, then the "roof" that "falls in" is representative of collapsing health. This medical metaphor is an early example of Yeats's attitude to death, that can be best matched with his figurative "conflagration in the rafters," which he uses to describe the near-death of Lady Gregory in his fiftieth journal entry on 4 February 1909 (*Autobiographies* 353). In his autobiographical collection of diary extracts from 1909 titled *Estrangement:*

Extracts From A Diary Kept In 1909 (1926), Yeats confides that Lady Gregory "brought to my wavering thoughts steadfast nobility" (*Autobiographies* 353). Deteriorating houses become a figurative pattern in Yeats's work from his early career, which shows an ever-present awareness of disintegrating health that is harmonised with space and place.

Yeats's dilapidated roof metaphor grows stronger at the turbulent points in his life, such as when Maud Gonne rejected his marriage proposal again in 1901 and when he almost loses Lady Gregory to illness in 1909. Gregory, his close friend and collaborator, suffered a suspected cerebral haemorrhage on 3 February 1909, although there are other potential diagnoses.[5] The kingfisher, whose "roof falls in of his tunnelled house" (book 1, line 423), belongs to *The Wanderings of Oisin* (1889). This is mirrored in the natural setting, as even the "fir-tree" that Oisin "smote" has a "leafless top" (lines 176–77). However, Yeats later adds his early-career metaphor to *The Countess Cathleen* (1892) in 1901, as the eponymous protagonist offers her home as a refuge for the victims of famine that "[m]ay escape from beak and claw; all, all shall come / Till the walls burst and the roof fall on us" (*VPl* lines 446–47).[6] These lines were first brought to life within the revised 1901 edition, where Yeats applied his roof as an extended metaphor in the same year as his rejected proposal. In order to save Irish people from famine, Countess Cathleen sacrifices her body, soul, medicines, and house. In Scene Two, she provides the ageing and ailing victims with protection in her own home. In Yeats's first edition

[5] Regarding Gregory's period of illness in 1909, Foster writes, "Though WBY carried on doggedly with his French lessons, his life was being taken over once more by everyday Dublin matters. And his health suffered. His smoking habit (adopted on and off through his life) had produced headaches and palpitations. Synge was back in hospital; WBY begged Gregory to come from Coole and help out. But surprise at her silence was replaced by severe chagrin and genuine consternation when Robert Gregory wrote on 4 February, telling him that she had herself been at death's door, having suffered a cerebral haemorrhage and—as she put it in a pencilled note—'nearly slipped away.' Robert's letter carried an implied rebuke about the 'excitement and worry' his mother had been subjected to, and told WBY that he and others would have to manage the theatre as best they could" (*The Apprentice Mage* 398). A New York Public Library note on this time states: "Drained by overwork, difficulties at the Abbey, and other worries, Gregory's health declined, leading to a nervous collapse and severe nosebleeds—often incorrectly described since as a cerebral hemorrhage—on February 3, 1909" ("A Friend's Illness").

[6] Unless otherwise stated, all the quotations for Yeats's plays are taken from *The Variorum Edition of the Plays of W. B. Yeats* (1966), edited by Russell K. Alspach and assisted by Catharine C. Alspach.

in 1892, titled *The Countess Kathleen and Various Legends and Lyrics*, Cathleen's imperative command is especially important as it engineers a purposeful wandering to safety and shelter, but there is no mention of the fragile roof: "Make no delay, / And bid them house here all the old and ailing" (44).[7] In his next two editions, in 1895 and 1899, Yeats left these lines undisturbed for the time being. *The Countess Cathleen* underwent a myriad of revisions since 1892, until the final draft was printed in 1912.[8] Yeats again reprinted his play in 1901, by which time Cathleen's imperative had fully evolved into:

> Come, follow me, for the earth burns my feet
> Till I have changed my house to such a refuge
> That the old and ailing, and all weak of heart,
> May escape from beak and claw; all, all, shall come
> Till the walls burst and the roof fall on us.
> From this day out I have nothing of my own. (*Poems* 52)

This was the last time that Yeats reconstructed Cathleen's imperative command and its surrounding semantics, as he kept these changes thereafter. Yeats's introduction of the roof, at a time of unrequited love, evidences a link between personal emotions and this figurative image. By extension, this extended metaphor peaks when Yeats applies the "conflagration in the rafters" to Gregory in 1909, thus linking her with Countess Cathleen (*Autobiographies* 353). Scholars, such as R. F. Foster, believe that the actress and republican revolutionary Maud Gonne was Yeats's muse when he created Cathleen as a character.[9] As Yeats dedicated his play to Gonne, it is likely that Gonne inspired his process of characterisation at the birth of his famine play, years before he first met Gregory at Lord Morris of Spiddal's party in London in 1894. As of 1909, however, it is evident that he suddenly assimilated Cathleen with Gregory more than Gonne. Not

[7] This is a reference to the first ever publication of *The Countess Kathleen*, as Yeats adapted these lines in later editions. This is the only edition where Yeats spells the eponymous protagonist's name as "Kathleen" instead of "Cathleen." The 1892 version of *The Countess Cathleen* is not divided into acts, but it is separated into five scenes.

[8] From 1892 to 1912, Yeats published seven revised editions of *The Countess Cathleen*. His last version, printed in 1912, was the one used in Abbey Theatre performances from 14 December 1911. Following this, the play was republished in more editions, but as an exact replica of the 1912 version.

[9] R. F. Foster states that Yeats's "meeting with Gonne helped inspire the image of an aristocratic beauty sacrificing herself for love of the people" (*Apprentice Mage* 97).

only does Yeats take his roof metaphor out of fiction and apply it to his ill friend through the "conflagration in the rafters" in 1909, Gregory also shares the qualities attributed to Cathleen, such as her attentiveness to health and support with both finance and emotional well-being. Gregory supported Yeats throughout their friendship.[10] Both Gregory and Cathleen provide metaphorical roofs of security, which serve as support systems that, when removed, risk holistic homelessness in mind and body. Cathleen fears that the roof will collapse, and the protection of her people would falter. Yeats almost loses his support system at the potential loss of Gregory. His extended metaphor, depicting a roofless home, lends itself to a compulsory wandering as the remedy for grief and a method with which to find a healthy coping mechanism and a new home for old memories.

The horror of age and how it is overcome is central to the poem, and Yeats's preoccupation with this fear ran throughout his entire career. Oisin, "sick with years," firstly overcomes elderly age with the "wandering dances" that "wound through the windless woods" on the immortal island, "[w]here men have heaped no burial-mounds" (book 1, lines 5, 275, 320, 82). He remembers that his "now outworn and withered hands" once held "some dead warrior's broken lance" (book 1, lines 349, 367). He "turned it in [his] hands" and "found in that forgetfulness" memories of "the blood-bedabbled plains" where "the Fenians stept" (lines 368, 365, 370–71). Niamh then "caught [his] hands, but spake no word / Save only many times [his] name" (lines 374–75). His "eyes grow dim" due to "all the ancient sorrow of men" and he is at the mercy of "ravening

[10] In both 1896 and 1897, Lady Gregory nursed Yeats back to health, whilst providing him with shelter at Coole House. This is explained in both Yeats's "Book V: The Stirring of the Bones" in *The Trembling of the Veil* (1922) and *Dramatis Personae 1896-1902* (1935) (*Autobiographies* 282–84, 298–99). R. F. Foster, however, notes in his article "Yeats and the Death of Lady Gregory" (2004) that "[a]s their lives progressed, the balance of exchange had reversed; with Yeats's advance to eminence and (comparative) financial security, he had been able to give succour, and a roof, to the increasingly impoverished Gregory on her visits to Dublin in the 1920s, just as she had done for him in his youth at Coole" (109). He then states, "But in her final illness, something like the old pattern reasserted itself" because "[f]rom the late summer of 1931, as Gregory's cancer inexorably advanced, Yeats once again made Coole rather than Dublin his home" (109). Foster writes, "Their relationship, as James Pethica has brilliantly demonstrated, had always been transactional—involving intellectual collaboration and emotional interdependence as well as financial loans and much hospitality" (109). See Pethica's chapter, "Patronage and Creative Exchange: Yeats, Lady Gregory and the Economy of Indebtedness," in *Yeats and Women* (1997), edited by Deirdre Toomey, for more information on Lady Gregory's financial help (168–204).

Sorrow" and "the hand of Wrath" (book 1, lines 380–81; book 2, 199). Although he becomes "weak and poor and blind, and lies / On the anvil of the world," this human experience has an antithetical effect (book 2, lines 203–04). We are told "[h]ow the hammers spring on the anvil, on the spearhead's burning spot" (book 3, line 83). Oisin's aged wandering is a sharpening and strengthening.

* * *

The Wanderings of Oisin and Other Poems (1889), the first book in which his epic poem appeared, marked an important point in both Yeats's literary development and that of the Irish Revival. At twenty-four years old, he brought this archetypal Revival poem into being.[11] Although he had published several books since 1885, Yeats identified the minute he started *The Wanderings of Oisin* in early 1887 as a point of conversion, where his writing became fully Irish. In the reflective notes belonging to his *Early Poems and Stories* (1925), Yeats declares, "Many of the poems in *Crossways*, certainly those upon Indian subjects or upon shepherds and fauns, must have been written before I was twenty, for from the moment I began *The Wanderings of Usheen*, which I did at that age, I believe, my subject matter became Irish" (527).[12] It is a salient point in the Irish Revival as some scholars, including Norreys J. O'Conor, date the Revival in Ireland to 1889.[13] The periodisation of the Irish Revival is somewhat of a contested terrain; its beginning is a grey area that hovers from 1889 to 1891. In *The Handbook of the Irish Revival* (2015), Declan Kiberd and P. J. Mathews contextualise the Revival as having "took place between 1891 and 1922"

[11] R. F. Foster states that the public "response" to the poem "vindicated" Yeats's "relentless efforts to carve out a niche in the literary world" and notes that he "had been working on the long narrative *The Wanderings of Oisin* from early in 1887 (mentioning the tale in an article, 'Fin Mac Cumhail,' for the *Gael* that April)" (*Apprentice Mage* 85, 81).

[12] "Crossways" was the name of a section in *Poems by W. B. Yeats* (1895). It includes much of the material from *The Wanderings of Oisin and Other Poems* (1889). In *A Commentary on the Collected Poems of W. B. Yeats* (1968), Norman Jeffares notes that the only two new additions to the collection printed in *Poems* (1895) were "The Ballad of Father O'Hart" and "The Ballad of the Foxhunter" (3).

[13] O'Conor, Norreys J. "Ireland's Literary Revival and Regional Writing." *The Georgia Review*, vol. 1, no. 4, 1947, pp. 420–26 (p. 420). O'Conor writes, "Of the various regional movements during the past fifty years, none has been more successful both in accomplishment and in attracting the attention of a non-regional audience than was the Irish Literary Revival between 1889 and the founding of the Irish Free State in 1922" (420).

(24). However, it is justifiable to claim that the birth of the Revival in Ireland was in 1889, the year that Yeats published *The Wanderings of Oisin*. Laura O'Connor's "W. B. Yeats and Modernist Poetry," a chapter published in *The Cambridge Companion to Irish Modernism* (2014), provides an effective way of dating the Irish Revival back to 1889. O'Connor writes that "Yeats's publishing career corresponds exactly with the c.1890-1939 periodization of modernism: Oscar Wilde favorably reviewed Yeats's *The Wanderings of Oisin* in 1889, and – at Yeats's request – 'Under Ben Bulben' was published in Irish newspapers after his death in 1939" (77).[14] Through the lens of modernism, an avant-garde and experimental literary movement that runs alongside Yeats's career, 1889 can be evidenced as the iconic year that marks the beginning of the Revival period.

The theme of "wandering" in Yeats's *The Wanderings of Oisin* is intrinsically medical, as it is a symptom that recovers the memories in the mind, and it is an attempt to revive a lost state. Oisin goes to the Land of Youth, which bestows eternal health and life upon him. When he leaves the undying lands, however, he is susceptible to injury on his travels. This becomes apparent after Oisin battles the demon and his "wounds" require healing "with unguents out of flowers" that are located "by some De Danaan shrine" (book 1, lines 185–86). Curative plants that grow in the west of Ireland include wheat, flowers, dandelions, and moss. Whilst medicine has the potential to restore declining patients, it is the countryside that grows and gives life to the herbs, thus acting as a natural practitioner of place. The roots of the Revival were always present in Irish soil, but it was Yeats who cultivated medicinal herbs into his written work, thereby making their health-giving properties more visible. He uprooted traditional Irish medicine, a significant part of Ireland's rural history, and applied it to a modern context in the hope that it would reconnect people to a sense of place and space that provides renewable medicine and an opportunity to heal from past wounds.

* * *

[14] In "W. B. Yeats and Modernist Poetry," O'Connor also states, "A Victorian and self-professed 'last Romantic' as well as a modernist, Yeats upsets the supposition that modernism constitutes a radical departure from what precedes it" (77).

Including the title, the word "wandering" and its variants occurs twenty-one times in *The Wanderings of Oisin*.[15] The poem has been the subject of a great deal of critical attention, and much emphasis has been placed on symbolic and historical perspectives it contains.[16] However, the use of "wandering" has not attracted critical attention, even though it appears prominently and was Yeats's own addition. Micheál Coimín (Michael Comyn; c. 1680–1760), an eighteenth-century Irish-language poet from County Clare, wrote *Laoi Oisín ar Tír na n-Óg* (*The Lay of Oisín in the Land of Youth*) in approximately 1750.[17] This Fenian tale of six hundred and thirty-six lines does not include this word at all. "Wandering," in English, is not just an adjective but a gerund. In Irish, *ag fánaíocht* means "wandering," which translates to the prepositional phrase "at roaming" in English. In the absence of gerunds, recognised by the syntactic unit and postmodifier "-ing," the Irish language uses non-finite verb forms for present participles.[18] In Irish, therefore, "wandering" can morph into an adjective, noun, verbal noun, or past or present participle. James Macpherson (1736–1796), the eighteenth-century Scottish poet who became notorious for promoting his own compositions as English versions

[15] This is a full concordance list for "wandering" in this epic poem: the titular "*The Wanderings of Oisin*," "wandering mind," "wandering moon," "the slow owls wandered," "wander away," "the wandering seas," "O Wandering Oisin," "wandering land breeze," "wandering hours," "merry wandering rout," "wandering dances," "the grey wandering osprey Sorrow" (repeated three times), "wandering ruby cars," "[s]ome wandered ever hand in hand," "wander singing," "wander in the storms and clinging snows," and "a wandering and milky smoke" (repeated three times) (p. 1; book 1, lines 2, 12, 41, 52, 55, 123, 165, 177, 253, 275, 303, 319, 342, 330, 389, 419; book 2, line 201; book 3, lines 1, 12, 148).

[16] Russell K. Alspach, Thomas R. Whitaker, and Michael J. Sidnell have conducted major Ossian studies. In "Some Sources of Yeats's 'The Wanderings of Oisin,'" Alspach focuses on Coimín's *Laoi Oisín ar Tír na n-Óg*, Middle Irish dialogue poetry, and selected English texts as influences for Yeats's *The Wanderings of Oisin* (849–50). In his article "The Early Yeats and the Pattern of History" (1960), Whitaker explores the tensions between Oisin and St. Patrick and therefore paganism and Christianity (320). In his article "The Allegory of Yeats's 'The Wanderings of Oisin'" (1979), Sidnell analyses the connection between imagery, symbolism, and allegory in Yeats's epic poem (139).

[17] Micheál Coimín (Michael Comyn) wrote the old Irish lyrical poem, *Laoi Oisín ar Tír na n-Óg* (*The Lay of Oisín in the Land of Youth*), in approximately 1750. Bryan O'Looney, Dáithí Coimín (David Comyn), and Tomás Ó Flannghaile (Thomas Flannery) respectively published the most famous translations of this lyrical poem in 1859, 1880, and 1896. Alspach believes that Yeats was most likely to have read O'Looney's translated edition ("Sources" 850).

[18] For more information on Irish grammar, see: Hickey, Raymond, "Features of Irish Syntax." *Lingua Posnaniensis*, vol. 26, 1985, pp. 15–26 (p. 8).

of the supposed Highland epic, *The Works of Ossian* (1765), does not include it in his Ossian and Fingal "translations" either.[19] For Yeats to have introduced this word and to have made it so central suggests its importance in his imagination.

The word "wandering" forms part of the initial description of the two lovers, Niamh and Oisin. Readers are told that the "wandering and milky smoke" that "[f]led foam underneath" and "round" the travelling Oisin and Niamh was as "[h]igh as the saddle-girth, covering away from [their] glances the tide" (book 3, lines 1–2). This smoke is far from being kin to the black miasmas that hung over the industrial cities of the nineteenth century. The word "milky" was known to mean "weak" from the early seventeenth century to the late twentieth century, but it also might indicate sustenance and nurturing ("milky"; *OED*). There is perhaps a relationship between the lack of forward momentum in *The Wanderings of Oisin* and the issue of wandering. This proposition persists in Yeats's work, such as in his poem "Tom O'Roughley" in *The Wild Swans at Coole* (1919) collection. In this poem, Tom O'Roughley says that "wisdom is a butterfly / And not a gloomy bird of prey," which is a variation on the theme of wandering (*VP* lines 7–8).

The process of wandering is central to the epic, but it is also important to the composition of the poem too. In his essay, "The Symbolism of Poetry" (1900), Yeats discusses the importance of a "wavering" rhythm:

> ... we would cast out of serious poetry those energetic rhythms, as of a man running, which are the invention of the will with its eyes always on something to be done or undone; and we would seek out those wavering, meditative, organic rhythms, which are the embodiment of the imagination, that neither desires nor hates, because it has done with time, and only wishes to gaze upon some reality, some beauty; nor would it be any longer possible for anybody to deny the importance of form, in all its kinds, for although you can expound an opinion, or describe a thing, when your words are not quite well chosen, you cannot give a body to something that moves beyond the senses, unless your words are as subtle, as complex, as full

[19] In *Early Bardic Literature, Ireland* (1879), Standish James O'Grady claims, "But MacPherson's Ossian is not a translation" (35). He expands, "In the publications of the Irish Ossianic poetry we see what that poetry really was—rude, homely, plain-spoken, leagues removed from the nebulous sublimity of MacPherson" (35).

of mysterious life, as the body of a flower … (*Essays and Introductions* 163–64)[20]

He treats composition as a skeletal frame designed to carry the flesh of symbolism. For example, anapestic hexameter carries the image of the wandering smoke that recurs three times in total. After the twice-repeated line "[f]led foam underneath us, and round us, a wandering and milky smoke," the "[h]alf open" eyes of the "king of the nails of gold" are described as "dull with the smoke of their dreams" (book 3, lines 1, 65, 61). When the "wandering and milky smoke" is repeated for the third time, it only encompasses the singular Oisin as it "[f]led foam underneath me, and round me" (line 148). The smoke, symbolic for ambiguity and pollution, occupies the same six feet per line but its meaning changes from a shared to an individual experience. It is a liminal boundary that separates Oisin and Niamh, health and illness, immortality and mortality, and forgetfulness and memory.

Yeats's friend, the doctor and poet Robert Bridges, championed this line from *The Wanderings of Oisin* because its prosaic rhythm captured his interest: "Fled foam underneath us, and round us, a wandering and milky smoke" (book 3, line 1). Bridges compliments the rhythm in this line as "a new thing in English poetry—Yeats made it—it was not there before" (qtd. in Sullivan 20). The line even made a humorous appearance in a letter to Yeats, where Bridges wrote of a train that "leaves Paddington at 6.10 and its wandering and milky smoke does not stop at Reading" (qtd. in Sullivan 20).[21]

At the time Yeats was writing, in the late nineteenth century, *vers libre* (free verse) was yet to surface and regular verse was still dominant.[22] However, it is debateable as to whether Yeats followed this trend, even

[20] "The Symbolism of Poetry" (April 1900) was first distributed in the sixth volume of *The Dome*, the aestheticist arts periodical. It was then reprinted in Yeats's collection of essays, *Ideas of Good and Evil*, published in 1903.

[21] In an invitation letter, Bridges asks Yeats if he would be willing to visit his home: "There is a very first class train from Paddington to Pangbourne of an evening. It leaves Paddington at 6.10 and its wandering and milky smoke does not stop at Reading" (qtd. in Sullivan 20). In "How Yeats Learned to Scan," Hannah Sullivan suggests that "[t]he very fact that Bridges was able to quote Yeats's phrase in a letter shows that it works in a natural prose sentence; there is nothing baroque or strained about it" (20).

[22] While free verse is present in France in the work of Jules Laforgue in the later nineteenth century, it does not appear in English-language poetry until the early twentieth century in the work of Ezra Pound and others.

though he penned some contrived lines that are strictly bound within iambic pentameter: "For a sign / I burst the chain: still earless, nerveless, blind, / Wrapped in the things of the unhuman mind" (lines 96–98). Hannah Sullivan, in her article titled "How Yeats Learned to Scan," attests that "[m]any critics write as if he occupied some nebulous middle ground between traditional form and free verse, and remained in the same metrical limbo for his entire career" (7). Sullivan argues, "By keeping the syntactic and the verse unit close, but just slightly off-kilter, Yeats forged a 'natural' style capable, at times, of pointed metrical artifice" (37). It is clear that Yeats did not completely conform to the literary climate, which was then dominated by regular verse, but he found his own tone and rhythm. Yeats's rhythm is a reference to wandering: it was not just a theme in the poem; it was a technique.

In his presentation of "wandering" as a positive, Yeats introduced a new element into the nascent Revival. Standish James O'Grady encouraged the Irish public to protect their heritage from extinction, and he advised them to be wary of Macpherson's translations, which were viewed as part of a false revival. O'Grady was described as the father of the Revival movement; *Early Bardic Literature, Ireland* (1879) also helped to inspire the Celtic Revival by popularising ancient legends. O'Grady emphasises that Irish literature is "not vague, nebulous, and shifting" (20). In the same foundational Revival text, he clarifies that Irish bards were not "loose wanderers," although he concedes that there were some "wandering undisciplined members" of the bardic organisation and class (50). "Wandering" is not something that O'Grady praises. Yeats would later subvert this negative perception of "wandering," as well as the role of the "wanderer," through the lens of folk cures and medicine.

* * *

Folk cures and medicine are present in the poem, such as "bowls of barley, honey, and wine," "oil and wine and honey and milk," "dewdrops," "the saffron morning," "the leaves of damask roses," the "drops of dew" that "in myriads fall," "unguents out of flowers," and "hazel and oak leaf" (book 1, lines 8, 92, 293, 277, 315, 222; book 2, line 185; book 3, line 23). It is important to note that Oisin ignores the monitory voice of St. Patrick who tells him that he is wrecked; his story is too strong to be stemmed. A strong story defies age. Patrick remarks that Oisin is "still wrecked among heathen dreams" (book 1, line 31). Oisin, however, ignores Patrick and continues speaking about his Fenian tales regardless of the interrupted narrative. Again, Oisin responds to Patrick with wandering when retelling Finn's conversation with Niamh. Fionn mac Cumhaill/ Finn MacCool, the legendary warrior and father to Oisin, speaks the following words that combat Patrick's statement about "heathen dreams":

> What dream came with you that you came
> Through bitter tide on foam-wet feet?
> Did your companion wander away
> From where the birds of Aengus wing? (book 1, lines 50–53)

This extended metaphor of the dream visually and orthographically crosses the boundaries on the page between Patrick's and Oisin's speech, and Niamh, as a character, goes beyond the geographical parameters between the immortal and mortal islands. Niamh's "dream," to marry Oisin, is more positive than the "heathen dreams" (book 1, line 31). When Finn asks Niamh if her "companion wander[ed] away / From where the birds of Aengus wing?" and awaits a response, Niamh reveals that she is also wandering in search of Oisin, about whom "the Danaan poets brought / Rhyme that rhymed upon Oisin's name" (lines 52–53, 63–64). Equally, her mind wanders too, as she becomes:

> ... dizzy with the thought
> Of all that wisdom and the fame
> Of battles broken by his hands,
> Of stories builded by his words. (book 1, lines 65–68)

It is Niamh who helps Oisin to triumph over the horror of age, as she brings Oisin to De Danaan lands "[w]here broken faith has never been known" (book 1, line 84). Oisin and Niamh "rode out from the human lands"; "Caoilte, Conan, and Finn came near, / And wept, and raised their lamenting hands" (lines 114, 111–12). This is reminiscent of "The Song of Wandering Aengus" (1897), a poem about the Celtic god of beauty and love who is travelling to find his beloved who "called [him] by [his] name" (line 12). Niamh similarly "named [Oisin] by sweet names," including "O Wandering Oisin" (book 2, line 27; book 3, line 123). In the later poem, republished in *The Wind Among the Reeds* in 1899, Aengus perseveres:

> Though I am old with wandering
> Through hollow lands and hilly lands,
> I will find out where she has gone,
> And kiss her lips and take her hands; ... (lines 17–20)

Written in iambic tetrameter, and thus interestingly the same metre as Book One of *The Wanderings of Oisin*, this poem begins with Aengus, who "went out to the hazel wood" (line 1). He "cut and peeled a hazel wand" in order to catch "a little silver trout," which metamorphosed into a "glimmering girl" who personally addressed him and then "faded through the brightening air" (lines 3, 8, 13, 16). This parallels lines from "The Stolen Child," such as the "wandering water" that "gushes / From the hills above Glen-Car" and the search for "slumbering trout" (lines 28–29, 32). The disappearance of the "glimmering girl" in "The Song of Wandering Aengus," rather like Oisin's longing to return to the Fenians, inspires Aengus's quest to

> ... walk among long dappled grass,
> And pluck till time and times are done
> The silver apples of the moon,
> The golden apples of the sun. (lines 21–24)

Similar to the "hazel wood" and "hazel wand," which lead to the magical and transformative encounter in "The Song of Wandering Aengus," Niamh tells the "O Wandering Oisin" that "the strength of the bell-branch is naught," which signifies magical access to the Tír na nÓg and contrasts with Patrick's "brazen bell" that carries connotations of Christianity (lines 1, 3; book 3, 123, 71).

Hazel is a type of wood, which was believed to have magical properties in Irish mythology. Far from "heathen dreams," "hazel and oak" appear three times in *The Wanderings of Oisin* (book 1, line 31; book 3, lines 10, 23, 25). Following the journey through the "wandering and milky smoke," Oisin asks a rhetorical question: "An isle lay level before us, with dripping hazel and oak?" (book 3, lines 1, 10). The horse, transporting them to each island, "gave a whinny; for, cumbrous with stems of the hazel and oak, / A valley flowed down from his hoofs" (lines 25–26). The "gleams of the world and the sun, / Ceased on our hands and our faces, on hazel and oak leaf" (lines 22–23). Although the eponymous Oisin's name is the focal point, Oisin instead anchors the Fenian appellations:

> As my mind made the names of the Fenians. Far from the hazel and oak,
> I rode away on the surges, where, high as the saddle-bow,
> Fled foam underneath me, and round me, a wandering and milky smoke.
> (lines 146–48)

Not only is the "hazel and oak" associated with the recurrent "wandering and milky smoke," it is also an environment that Oisin geographically moves away from and therefore rejects. Lady Jane Wilde writes that hazel is one of the "most sacred trees in Ireland" and that "St. Patrick drove out the serpents from Ireland" using "a hazel wand" (*Ancient Cures* 56). Within old Irish superstition, it is reported that "with a hazel stick a person can draw a circle round himself, within which no evil thing can enter—fairy, or demon, or serpent, or evil spirit" on the condition that the stick is "cut on May morning, and before sunrise, to make it powerful" (Wilde, *Ancient Cures* 57). Oisin drives himself away "[f]ar from the hazel and oak," and from any chance of returning to the Tír na nÓg, which is symbolised by the diminishing power of the bell-branch (line 146). Just as St. Patrick expels the serpents from Ireland, and entraps one in Killarney's Great Lake, Oisin drives out the negative perceptions of the Fenians and the forgetfulness that had befallen the ancient legends.

Wandering is a medical weakness, associated with age and decrepitude, which can be tracked in the three books that constitute *The Wanderings of Oisin*. From the outset, it is a prototype for infirmity and senescence that first appears in Oisin's dialogue with St. Patrick in Book One: "You who are bent, and bald, and blind, / With a heavy heart and a wandering mind" (lines 1–2). The form in which these lines are written, in monosyllabic tetrameter, animates a steady pace that manifests the impending age that is incumbent upon Oisin. The alliterative plosives, "bent, and bald, and blind," create a sound reminiscent of a beating drum or a ticking clock, counting down Oisin's remaining years on earth. Alternatively, the regular rhythm represents a stable heartbeat that later becomes arrhythmic as the form wanders away, thus representing a body losing its reliable health. The "heavy heart" and the "wandering mind" are symbols, encased within the trochaic structure, that support the palpitating rhythm that is plagued with atrial fibrillation (faster heartbeats) and bradycardia (slower heartbeats).

In terms of medicine in the twenty-first century, "wandering" is classified as a symptom of memory and dissociative disorders (Andrews 322; Martin 216). Long before Yeats's lifetime, however, it was well established that this term referred to the "uncontrolled" movement of the "mind, thoughts, [and] desires" ("Wander"; *OED*). According to the *Google Books Ngram Viewer*, a linguistic computer programme that plots word frequency based on a substantial corpus, the usage of "wandering" peaked in English fiction in 1874 ("Wandering"; Orwant and Brockman). Other contemporary writers were using "wandering" in a negative sense, such as the Irish poet Sir Charles Gavan Duffy in his *The Ballad Poetry of Ireland* (1845). Re-published in the same year as the usage of "wandering" peaked, Duffy's manuscript also holds a place in Yeats's own library.[23] Duffy uses "wandering" negatively to denote "wandering far" from home, to lament "memory" that "is wandering back to long departed years" that proceeds a "heavy" heart and "eyes" that "are full of tears," and to describe "[a]n 'alien,' an outcast, a wandering slave" (51, 73, 141). In Charles Dickens's *Great Expectations* (1861), "wandering" is presented as a restless state in so far as the protagonist is endowed with a triadic structure that emphasises his attachment to "that staid old house near the Green at Richmond": "Let my body be where it would, my spirit was always wandering, wandering, wandering, about that house" (299). Loaded with negative connotations, this popular word was present in the discourse of Victorian society and famous writers, which means that Yeats would have been familiar with its relationship to medical decline and debilitation.

Yeats wishes to associate wandering with renewed resourcefulness and strength. This turning point occurs after the heroic Oisin rescued the incarcerated woman and defeated the demon, when Niamh and the unnamed captive healed his battle injuries whilst being "[f]ull of hope and dread":

> Those two came carrying wine and meat and bread,
> And healed my wounds with unguents out of flowers
> That feed white moths by some De Danaan shrine; ... (book 2, lines 183–86)

It is possible that Yeats is referring to the famous herbal legend that surrounds the De Danaan physicians. This ancient account is covered in Lady Jane Wilde's *Ancient Cures, Charms, and Usages of Ireland* (1890). Originally, this folk tale is anonymously penned in the sixteenth-century

[23] Duffy's 1874 edition of *The Ballad Poetry of Ireland* is listed in Edward O'Shea's *A Descriptive Catalog of W. B. Yeats' Library* (1985) because it holds a place in Yeats's library (O'Shea 85; Duffy, MS 40,568/77).

Cath Maige Tuired: The Second Battle of Mag Tuired, which contains material from much earlier periods.[24] Wilde's retelling of this manuscript's medical section chimes with Yeats's "unguents out of flowers" and the "De Danaan shrine" that intervals Oisin's wanderings. Much like the flowers that are administered to Oisin's wounds after his battle with the demon, Wilde describes the "historic battle of Moytura" and how "Dianecht, the chief physician of the Tuatha, had a bath of herbs prepared, at the rear of the army, of singular efficacy, into which the wounded were plunged, and from which they emerged healed and whole" (*Ancient Cures* 6). This same hereditary physician created "a silver hand" for "Nuada, the King of the Tuatha" who "lost his hand" in the fight (Wilde, *Ancient Cures* 6).[25] Yeats writes the healing moment, when Oisin's battle wounds are absolved with herbs, as a continuation of De Danaan medicine: "The sons were generally educated by their fathers in the practice of physic, but it is said that Dianecht, being jealous of the superior skill of his son, caused him to be slain, when from the grave of the youth sprang a number of herbs, all efficacious in curing disease; and thus, though dead, he carried on his work" (Wilde, *Ancient Cures* 8). This emanation of herbs from the grave is reminiscent of Yeats's "De Danaan shrine," from where the flowers are found so that unguents could be extracted from them and applied to Oisin's wounds. Just as Niamh and the rescued woman are employed to select the herbs, this role is also attributed to a female character in *Cath Maige Tuired: The Second Battle of Mag Tuired*. It is Airmed, the goddess of herbal medicine and Míach's sister, who is responsible for continuing the healing tradition:

[24] Gerard Murphy states that the *Cath Maige Tuired* (*The Battle of Mag Tuired*) is "the product of an eleventh or twelfth-century redactor working mainly upon ninth-century material" ("Notes on *Cath Maige Tuired*" 195). Elizabeth A. Gray provides a translation, from Irish to English, of *Cath Maige Tuired: The Second Battle of Mag Tuired*. The reference for the sixteenth-century manuscript is: British Library, London, Harleian MS 5280, fols. 63a–70b (*Cath Maige Tuired*; Harleian MS 5280).

[25] In Elizabeth A. Gray's translation of *Cath Maige Tuired: The Second Battle of Mag Tuired*, it is written that Míach (Dían Cécht's son) "went to the hand [of Núadu] and said 'joint to joint of it, and sinew to sinew'" and healed it "in nine days and nights" (33). In jealousy, Dían Cécht "hurled a sword at the crown of his son's head and cut his skin to the flesh" (33). Having been attacked three times, Míach heals himself after every wound. However, the fourth attack "cut out the brain, so that Míach died; and Dían Cécht said that no physician could heal him of that blow" (33).

> After that, Míach was buried by Dían Cécht, and three hundred and sixty-five herbs grew through the grave, corresponding to the number of his joints and sinews. Then Airmed spread her cloak and uprooted those herbs according to their properties. Dían Cécht came to her and mixed the herbs, so that no one knows their proper healing qualities unless the Holy Spirit taught them afterwards. And Dían Cécht said, "Though Míach no longer lives, Airmed shall remain." (Gray, *Cath Maige Tuired* 33)

Yeats's aim, using De Danaan herbs and magic in his writing, is to revive an ailing Irish heritage that can survive in a new modern world. Wilde paraphrases a section of an anonymous poem that appears in *The Book of Invasions* and speaks to Yeats's vision for Ireland:

> The Tuatha by force of potent spells,
> Could raise a slaughtered army from the earth,
> And make them live, and breathe, and fight again. (*Ancient Cures* 6)

Although Yeats's lines about the "unguents out of flowers" are written in iambic pentameter, polysyndeton is a similarity that wanders throughout all three books, particularly in the speech that he assigns to Oisin. He refers to himself as "bent, and bald, and blind" in Book One, which morphs into "weak and poor and blind" in the second book (book 1, line 1; book 2, line 203). However, *in media res*, the polysyndeton entertains the more positive and celebratory "wine and meat and bread," which accompanies the floral ointment (book 2, line 184). The flowers are collected before "the sun once more in saffron stept," which is important because the morning dew is a healing property in itself that contributes to herbal remedies (line 192). Oisin's healing therefore appears to fit within this traditional time frame and allows him to again "wander in the storms and clinging snows" (line 201). Niamh's role in the epic should not be underestimated: she is the bridge between the mortal and immortal lands, between hurting and healing, between illness and health, and therefore between being stationary and continuing to wander.

Yeats uses a wandering rhythm to restore Ireland and give a new definition to "wandering." The ailments, which come upon Oisin in Book Three, are part of the wandering that returns his beating heart back to Ireland. Despite the irregularity of the anapestic hexameter, mimicking a murmuring and arrhythmic heartbeat, Oisin has restored Ireland's body: "Not coughing, my head on my knees, and praying, and wroth with the bells" becomes "[a]h me! to be shaken with coughing and broken with old age and pain" (book 3, lines 159, 217). In physiological lexicon, "wandering" pain moves around the body and the aetiology is often unknown ("Wandering"; *OED*). The polysyndetic list, "to be shaken with coughing and broken with old age and pain," is elongated with added anapestic feet that are suggestive of a wandering health. Both Oisin's geographical travels and his migratory symptoms, from being "bent, and bald, and blind" to becoming "shaken" and "broken," are necessary for the Irish past to be fixed into a settled abode within the present and future.

The antithesis between "coughing" and "not coughing" marks a metamorphosis from health to illness for Oisin's body. For his soul and sense of self, however, he forgets and then remembers his Irish past, and he therefore moves from a state of losing his identity to finding it again. This rediscovery has resounding implications on Ireland as a nation as Oisin's stories, rehoused in their native country, secure the roots and foundations of Irish heritage. Yeats does not commit to a prescriptive prosody, but he writes his own spontaneous prescription for each poem, and he therefore preserves his own literary health and freedom. The sporadic waning and wandering rhythm embodies and imitates medical frailty, connected with declining age and deterioration.

Old age and decay versus youth are a central theme for Yeats and Oisin. He mentions the elixir of life no less than five times in his autobiographies, which indicates his awareness of the encroachment of old age.[26] This means that both Yeats and his character experience wandering as a preservation of life and memory. Whereas he realises that death is necessary for new life, Yeats is preoccupied with avoiding decay and decrepitude. In "Book I: Four Years: 1887-1891" (1921) of his autobiography *The Trembling of the Veil* (1922), Yeats describes a meeting with "an old white-haired Oxfordshire clergyman," who talks about witnessing an apparition in his "alchemical laboratory in a cellar under my house" (*Autobiographies* 160). The subsequent passage is a response to Yeats's question about his success in alchemical research:

> "Yes, I once made the elixir of life. A French alchemist said it had the right smell and the right colour" (the alchemist may have been Eliphas Levi, who visited England in the 'sixties, and would have said anything [Yeats's

[26] Yeats mentions the philosophers' stone on three occasions in his autobiographies (*Autobiographies* 162, 265, 396).

> words]), "but the first effect of the elixir is that your nails fall out and your hair falls off. I was afraid that I might have made a mistake and that nothing else might happen, so I put it away on a shelf. I meant to drink it when I was an old man, but when I got it down the other day it had all dried up." (160)

The references to preservation of life do not stop at this passage. Yeats brings the author and occultist MacGregor Mathers, formerly known as Liddell Mathers, into his discussion about the elixir:

> He was a necessary extravagance, and he had carried further than any one else a claim implicit in the romantic movement from the time of Shelley and of Goethe; and in body and in voice at least he was perfect; so might Faust have looked in his changeless aged youth. In the credulity of our youth we secretly wondered if he had not met with, perhaps even been taught by, some old man who had found the elixir. Nor did he undeceive us. "If you find the elixir," he was accustomed to say, "you always look a few years younger than the age at which you found it. If you find it at sixty you will look fifty for a hundred years." None of us would have admitted that we believed in stone or elixir, the old Oxfordshire clergyman excited no belief, yet one among us certainly laboured with crucible or athanor. (162)

It is important to investigate Yeats's memories of the years in which he was composing his Revivalist poem, as these remembrances show that an "O wandering Yeats" accompanies an "O wandering Oisin" (book 3, line 123).

* * *

The word "wandering" is used so frequently that it becomes a keynote (as well as being in the title). The "grey wandering Osprey sorrow" depicts a bird that hunts for its prey (book 1, lines 303, 319, 342). The dancers are likened to a "merry wandering rout," and the stars have "wandering ruby cars" (book 1, lines 253, 330). Of the Immortals, "[s]ome wandered ever hand in hand"; other unfortunates, Oisin reflects, "wander in the storms and clinging snows" (book 1, line 389; book 2, line 201). Metaphorically, the "trumpet-twisted shell" is personified as sleeping "in immortal silence" and "[d]reaming of her own melting hues, / Her golds, her ambers, and her blues" (book 1, lines 160–63). This mixing and blending of colours foreground the "wandering land breeze" that accompanies "a far sound of feathery quires" that "seemed to blow from the dying flame" (lines 165–67). This is an otherworld where "purpose drifts and dies"; another island is enwreathed with “a wandering and milky smoke”; he is addressed by Niamh as “O wandering Oisin” (book 2, line 244; book 3, lines 1, 12, 148, 123). *The Wanderings of Oisin* as a whole, with the amalgamating colours of “golds,” “ambers,” and “blues,” is a Pre-Raphaelite painting in poem form. This Pre-Raphaelite Brotherhood was a nineteenth-century movement that was based on paintings and anti-materialistic ideas. Yeats’s *The Wanderings of Oisin* is a poem on canvas that speaks into the wider European movement.

Wandering was a restorative framework for action. Whereas, the Industrial Revolution (1760–1840) created men and machines that could not wander. This was a preoccupation of the London-born William Morris, a textile designer, literary artist, and the editor for the *Commonweal* journal, to which Yeats made contributions. Morris opposed English industrialism, as he saw first-hand that people working in Victorian England were dehumanised, overworked, and treated like cogs in a machine. Morris’s influence is encapsulated in his essay, *The Aims of Art* (1887), where he addressed a shared humanity. He writes about the contentious moods of energy and idleness in relation to industrialisation and working environments. For example: “when the mood of idleness is on me I find it hard indeed if I cannot rest and let my mind wander over the various pictures, pleasant or terrible, which my own experience or my communing with the thoughts of other men, dead or alive, have fashioned in it,” and he undergoes “a period of pain” if “circumstances will not allow me to cultivate this mood of idleness” (Morris 4). He saw that work was crushing and torturing people, and he wanted to re-embrace mediaeval artisanal freedom and creativity in contemporary England: he believed that mediaeval creativity could restore humanity.

Morris’s rejection of Victorian materialism links to Yeats’s wish to inaugurate a new era that would reject both the rationalism of the eighteenth century and the materialism of the nineteenth century. In his essay, Morris argues that there was an “Artificial Famine, caused by men working for the profit of a master” and that “the aim of art was to destroy the curse of labour” (32, 26). He predicted that “the ‘Aims of Art’ will be realised, though I know that they cannot be, so long as we groan under the tyranny of Artificial Famine” and warns his readers “against supposing, you who may specially love art, that you will do any good by attempting to revivify art by dealing with its dead exterior” (Morris 37–38). Yeats wanted a new, independent Ireland; Morris wanted a re-born England. Yeats had nationalistic ideas, such as Ireland becoming self-governing. He thought that society was too rational and materialistic, and he used materials and legends to pave the way for a newer and freer future, and as a rejection of Victorian utilitarianism and industrialisation. Irish mythological wandering, like Morris's mediaeval artisanal creativity, could restore humanity. Yeats is not engineering a narrow nationalism, but is working in a wider spiritual, cultural, social, and intellectual project.

The poem reaches a rhetorical high point in the promises of Niamh: this is the treasure wandering can bring. This is not to any destination or grail but "Danaan leisure" (book 1, line 100). At this point, Oisin disappears with Niamh to the various islands, and she promises that he "shall know the Danaan leisure" (line 100). Using a semi-colon, Yeats attaches this vow to "Niamh be with [him] for a wife" (line 101). Niamh is the conciliator between human and immortal life, and she plans to remain in immortal paradise "when the white moon climbs, / The red sun falls and the world grows dim" (lines 104–05). Niamh mentions a treasure—the "Danaan leisure"—that ironically grows to enhance Oisin's "ancient sadness of man," his desire to "leave the Immortals, their dimness, their dews dropping sleep," and his realisation that "twilight and slumber were gone" (book 1, line 100; book 3, lines 107–08, 112). Paradoxically, wandering is Yeats's purpose: it offers something restorative to a mechanised and fallen world. Yeats is not only referring to Irish nationalism and his desire for the self-governance of Ireland. He was not just engaged in Irish nationalist ideas; he was also speaking to other nationalities. Yeats wanted a new phase of human existence, which was part of a wider epochal change.

Morris believed in the ethic of leisure, and the restorative and necessary nature of taking time off, as opposed to a Victorian culture that fostered the utilitarian belief that there was no way of valuing or celebrating recreation. Both Yeats and Morris employ Niamh's wisdom of leisure, and they both tend to similar ethics. This is reminiscent of Keats's "negative capability," which is the belief that people should not ask questions, but instead try to be useful (*Poetical Works and Letters* 277). The Arthurian legends are a search for the Holy Grail, but *The Wanderings of Oisin* is much less utilitarian because it is a quest for "Danaan leisure." Niamh is not merely an accessory or auxiliary to the wanderings, but she is a female Oisin who is key to the protagonist crossing the boundary to the mortal lands, growing old again through wandering, and ultimately saving Ireland and the world. Niamh takes part in Oisin's debilitation of the body but also in the rehabilitation of Ireland.

Yeats was a new Romantic, reflecting the vision of Romanticism. The chasm is between Oisin's desire to know as opposed to Niamh's insistence for incertitude. This exemplifies the poet John Keats's concept of "negative capability," which is the power to not know or take in the knowledge of the great poets, but rather to foster the ability to exist without certainty (277). This Romantic mindset is epitomised in Keats's letter to his brothers, George and Thomas Keats, which was dated on 22 December 1817: "[A]t once it struck me what quality went to form a Man of Achievement, especially in Literature, and which Shakspeare [sic] possessed so enormously—I mean *Negative Capability*, that is, when a man is capable of being in uncertainties, mysteries, doubts, without any irritable reaching after fact and reason" (277). Oisin, like a Romantic, is being schooled in negative capability. He is part of an intellectual wandering; he is not tied down by structure as it is another world that he is negating.

Oisin's attempts to obtain data from Niamh, through his question as to whether the figures he sees are human or fairy, are dismissed. This is intellectual wandering. Oisin sees "a lady" that "rode like the wind / With an apple of gold in her tossing hand" and "a beautiful young man" who "followed behind / With quenchless gaze and fluttering hair" (book 1, lines 142–45). On asking the interrogative, "Were these two born in the Danaan land, / Or have they breathed the mortal air?" and therefore requesting an answer, Niamh replies with an imperative command to "[v]ex them no longer" (lines 146–48). Yeats uses anaphora to describe that Niamh does not wish to find this missing information: "And sighing bowed her gentle head, / And sighing laid the pearly tip / Of one long finger on my lip" in order to re-enact the mundane and monotonous repetition of "Danaan leisure" as opposed to Oisin's curiosity and inquisition (lines 149–51, 100). "Wandering" means not travelling with any purpose ("Wandering"; *OED*). Niamh is offering experience rather than a destination. Oisin, however, begins with a search for knowledge, which Niamh discourages.

* * *

The revival would bring about a new way of seeing the world, and Yeats added a framing to the restorative wandering of the spirit and to a debilitated present-day Ireland. In his essay "The Celtic Element in Literature" (1898), Yeats envisions a new world that is free from the shackles of rationalism and materialism:

> The reaction against the rationalism of the eighteenth century has mingled with a reaction against the materialism of the nineteenth century, and the symbolical movement, which has come to perfection in Germany in Wagner, in England in the Pre-Raphaelites, in France in Villiers de l'Isle-Adam, and Mallarmé, and in Belgium in Maeterlinck, and has stirred the imagination of Ibsen and D'Annunzio, is certainly the only movement that is saying new things. (*Essays and Introductions* 187)[27]

This departure from rationalist and materialist thought leads to a wandering towards Romanticism, nature, and emotion. In his conclusion to "The Celtic Element in Literature," Yeats compliments Slavonic, Finnish, Scandinavian, Welsh, and Greek legends (187). Utilising the role of Oisin as the questioner, he draws from old, well-known material with a new and invigorating approach. He resolves that "the Irish legends move among known woods and seas, and have so much of a new beauty that they may well give the opening century its most memorable symbols" (187). This is best demonstrated by his own questions on seeking and finding the unknown from the known:

> Oisin, new come from his three hundred years of faeryland, and of the love that is in faeryland, bids Saint Patrick cease his prayers a while and listen to the blackbird, because it is the blackbird of Derrycarn that Finn brought from Norway, three hundred years before, and set its nest upon the oak-tree with his own hands. Surely if one goes far enough into the woods, one will find there all that one is seeking? Who knows how many centuries the birds of the woods have been singing? (179)

Yeats associated wandering with a new mystical and spiritual epoch; it was a rejection of the predetermined courses of rationalism and materialism.

So, this is not just wandering for its own sake, it was, as Seamus Heaney astutely remarked, "a conscious counter-cultural act against the rationalism and materialism of late Victorian England" (*Finders Keepers* 99). In Book Two of *The Wanderings of Oisin*, "wandering" is valued more than "leisure" (book 1, lines 2, 100). Before Oisin battles the demon, he describes the "[w]indowless, pillarless, multitudinous home / Of faces" that "waited; and the leisured gaze / Was loaded with the memory of days

[27] Yeats's essay, "The Celtic Element in Literature," was first published in *Cosmopolis* in June 1898, an international literary magazine that was distributed on a monthly basis. It was then reprinted in Yeats's later compilation of essays, *Ideas of Good and Evil* (1903).

/ Buried and mighty" (book 2, lines 148–51). Oisin also remembers a "demon's leisure" in the form of "eyes, first white, now burned / Like wings of kingfishers; and he arose / Barking" (lines 168–70). The shape-shifting and metamorphic nature of this demon that "ran / Through many shapes" defies both restrictive materialism and rational thought (lines 174–75). The "new-healed shape" of the "dull and unsubduable" demon could only come into fruition when "at the sundown" Oisin "threw him in the surge, / To lie until the fourth morn saw emerge" (lines 221, 217, 219–20). Yeats's *The Wanderings of Oisin* is an intrinsic "new-healed shape" that has been liberated from rationalism and materialism.

Yeats took a mystical view of the future of humanity, which links to his refusal of utilitarianism and the clock. "Wandering" is an antiserum to Victorian utilitarianism: Oisin has "hands that hold no wearisome tool" (book 1, lines 340). In the song to the stars that have "wandering ruby cars," Oisin and the De Danaan sing about their opinion that these stars are "rul[ed] ... with an iron rod" and held "with an iron bond" (lines 330, lines 332–33). Yeats's indirect arguments against philosopher John Stuart Mill's (1806–1873) *Utilitarianism* (1879), the belief in the greatest good for the most substantial quantity of people, emerge with an anaphora: "Each one woven to the other, / Each one woven to his brother" (lines 334–35). Although Yeats uses a simile to compare this individual and societal dependency to being "[l]ike bubbles in a frozen pond," he ensures that his character remembers that "we in a lonely land abide / Unchainable as the dim tide, / With hearts that know nor law nor rule" (lines 336–39). Oisin is "[f]olded in love that fears no morrow, / Nor the grey wandering osprey Sorrow" (lines 341–42). Yeats is reclaiming "wandering" from being a medical sign of weakness to a restorative wandering of the spirit and to a debilitated present-day Ireland.

By reading William Blake's works, Yeats absorbed the conviction that there is no growth without controversy. In *The Marriage of Heaven and Hell* (1794), William Blake states that "[w]ithout contraries is no progression" and "[a]ttraction and repulsion, reason and energy, love and hate, are necessary to human existence" (7). By extension, therefore, health and illness can be added to this list as both strength and pain are at the heart of the human life and condition. In "The Municipal Gallery Revisited" (1937), an elegiac poem that remembers both people and happenings in Yeats's lifetime, he seeks to redefine "[t]he dead Ireland of my youth" as "an Ireland / The poets have imagined, terrible and gay" (lines 11–12). In the 1916 Rising, there was the birth of a terrible beauty, as described in the refrain that is repeated three times in Yeats's poem "Easter 1916" (1921): "A terrible beauty is born" (lines 16, 40, 80). Yeats was thinking in antithetical terms. By reading William Blake's works, he is taught to view the world with the lens that there is no growth without controversy. He begins to view death and ageing not as an end, but as a beginning. Yeats's status as the apprentice in the Revival had gone as he became a significant Revival figure.

* * *

The Countess Cathleen (1892) is a famine play, whereby the eponymous heroine is a patron responsible for her tenants "*in Ireland and in old times*" (3). Due to a time of famine in Ireland, the tenants are starving and sacrifice their souls in exchange for gold. Other characters that feature in this play include Aleel, a poet with a "wounded hand," that again recalls Núadu's injured hand and Míach's cure in *Cath Maige Tuired: The Second Battle of Mag Tuired* (sc. 3, line 527). Cathleen provides her tenants with grain, cattle, shelter, medicines, and then, ultimately, sacrifices her own soul so that the souls of her people "must be set free" (sc. 5, line 805). At the resolution, her sinful act is forgiven, and she is given access to Heaven. *The Wanderings of Oisin* (1889) is widely recognised as the birth of the Irish Renaissance. *The Countess Cathleen*, similarly, "marked the beginning of the Irish Revival in the theatre" when "the play was first performed in Dublin in 1899" (Drabble et al., *Concise Oxford Companion* 159). Both *The Wanderings of Oisin* and *The Countess Cathleen*, apart from the fact that they include physical and spiritual illness, are Yeats's initial treatments that ironically begin a national and universal healing process in literature.

In the context of a period of famine in Ireland, the herbs in *The Countess Cathleen* (1892) were an organic salve, much like the "unguents out of flowers" that healed Oisin's wounds (book 2, line 185). Even though "[t]he treasure-room is broken in" and "[t]he door stands open, and the gold is gone," the real treasure is the medicines that are stored in the "small room" (sc. 3, lines 623–24, 591). In *The Wanderings of Oisin*, Niamh's promise is the "Danaan leisure"; Countess Cathleen's gift is the herbal medicine that she provides for the peasants (book 1, line 100). In Scene Four, Cathleen leads a dialogue between a peasant, a porter, and foster-mother Oona. She is mindful that "[w]hen we meet again / I may have grown forgetful" (lines 646–47). She gives the peasant, who has experience in animal medicine, access to her herb collection:

> But take you this. It opens the small room
> Of herbs for medicine—of helebore,
> Of vervain, monkshood, plantain, and self-heal,
> And all the others; and the book of cures
> Is on the upper shelf. You understand
> Because you doctored goats and cattle once. (lines 591–96)

When the porter asks why she gave away her medicines, intimating that this was because she could "see / [Her] coffin in a dream" and then finds out that "[t]he treasure-room is broken in" and "[t]he door stands open, and the gold is gone," Cathleen makes some famine-related comments at the end of Scene Three. She states that "[a] sad resolve wakes in me. I have heard / A sound of wailing in unnumbered hovels" (sc. 3, lines 599–600). She then says, "Pray for the poor folk who are crazed with famine" (line 602). Echoes of the Irish Famine (1845–1852) are entwined with the mentions of medicine.

The first two cures in Yeats's list of cures, "helebore" and "vervain," are adjacently placed in the exact same order and on the same page in Wilde's *Ancient Cures, Charms, and Usages of Ireland* (39–40). This enchiridion of folk remedies was published in 1890, just two years before Yeats released *The Countess Cathleen* in 1892. As Yeats owned a copy of Wilde's book in his library, it is likely that he gleaned from it his knowledge of traditional medicine that presents itself in the early drafts of the play. The "book of cures" in *The Countess Cathleen*, containing information about "herbs for medicine" that are offered up to alleviate the "sound of wailing in unnumbered hovels," is located "on the upper shelf." Yeats may have had his own library shelves in mind when he wrote these lines and, by extension, Wilde's collection of natural remedies. For the 1895 edition of *The Countess Cathleen* in *Poems*, Yeats excised his list of cures from the play, but he re-employed them in the next edition in 1899. It is interesting that he removes the traditional herbs fourteen years before Gregory's near-death in 1909, as this is a dress rehearsal for when he abandons folk health-care and resorts to conventional medicine after her passing in 1932.[28] His tendency to rely on Wilde's work for medical information perhaps

[28] On 5 or 6 April 1934, near the anniversary of Gregory's death that happened two years before on 22 May 1932, Yeats relied upon the Steinach Operation in order to improve his health.

prompted him to cut out any specific links back to the healing book that informed much of his material.

Through paraphrasing, Wilde lists hellebore and vervain in the same chronology as Thomas Joseph Pettigrew, a surgeon living between the seventeenth and eighteenth centuries, whose antiquarian tastes led to him writing *On Superstitions Connected with the History and Practice of Medicine and Surgery* in 1843 (Wilde 39–40; Pettigrew 39). In his collection of medical superstitions, Pettigrew states:

> Black hellebore was to be plucked, not cut, and this with the right hand, which was then to be covered with a portion of the robe, and secretly conveyed to the left hand. The person gathering it was also to be clad in white, to be barefooted, and to offer a sacrifice of bread and wine.[29] Verbena or vervain was to be gathered at the rising of the dog-star, when neither sun nor moon shone, an expiatory sacrifice of fruit and honey having been previously offered to the earth. Hence arose its power to render the possessor invulnerable, to cure fevers, to eradicate poison, and to conciliate friendship. (39)

The black hellebore, gathered before dawn, is reminiscent of Oisin's "unguents out of flowers" that were also administered alongside "wine and meat and bread" (book 2, lines 184–85). Honey, accessory to the vervain herb, parallels "[t]he wild-bee's honey" at the start of Scene Two in *The Countess Cathleen* (line 292). It is likely that Yeats had read Wilde's work on healing prior to his composition of *The Countess Cathleen*, which influenced his material that specialises in herbal medicine.

In folk medicine, the five herbs that feature in these lines were once thought to either resist infection or remove negative substances from the body or could negatively be used as poisons.[30] Yeats's works, particularly

[29] At this point, Pettigrew includes Roman author Gaius Plinius Secundus, known as Pliny the Elder, in a footnote that reads: "Plinii Hist. Nat., lib. xxiv. c. 11" (39).

[30] Culpeper notes that the bark of hellebore roots was an ingredient for a syrup that was thought to have properties that "purge[s]" and "resist[s]" (307). Wilde states that "[v]ervain and the mountain ash are the best preservatives for cattle against witchcraft" (34). If "[s]ome should be tied round the cow's horns and her tail," then "no fairy or witch can do harm while the herbs of power are on her" (Wilde 34). Culpeper writes that vervain "kills and expels worms in the belly" and "helps the cough, wheezings, and shortness of breath, and all the defects of the reins and bladder, expelling the gravel and stone" (187–188). Furthermore, Culpeper writes that the plantain herbs are "good wound herbs" (142).

his epic poem and famine play, achieve a metaphorical cleansing and self-healing against false revivals, exterior influences, and being forgotten. Being internationalist in approach, he boosts the Irish immune system so that the public mind does not forget the past, which is represented in his selection of illness-resisting herbs. Wilde notes that, in ancient Ireland, "poison was extracted from hellebore" because warriors used "poisoned weapons" (255). The seventeenth-century herbalist and botanist Nicholas Culpeper (1616–1654) notes that "the bark of black [h]ellebore roots six drams" was an ingredient for a syrup that was thought to have properties that "purges melancholy" and "resists madness" (307).

Vervain was used to "cure fevers, to eradicate poison, and to conciliate friendship" (Pettigrew 39). The nineteenth-century physician Thomas Duché Mitchell (1791–1865) writes about monkshood, which was also known as aconite. He states that "although the [aconite] leaf is decidedly poisonous, it loses that property, by long ebullition" (82). He claims that "[t]he therapeutic properties of aconite and aconitina are, *anodyne, sedative, diaphoretic, diuretic*," and that "[p]hysicians, in former times, employed aconite in *gout, rheumatism, … cancers, epilepsy, palsy, dropsy*" and other conditions (Mitchell 83). James Cullen, an informant in *The Schools' Manuscript Collection* (*NFCS*), where students across the Republic of Ireland gathered folklore for the *National Folklore Collection* (*NFC*) from their neighbours and family members in the 1930s, states that "[t]he plaintain (slánlus) is used for stopping bleeding, especially the bleeding from a cut leg, hand or finger" ("Local Cures" 233).[31] This medicine would have been applicable to Aleel's "wounded hand" in *The Countess Cathleen* (sc. 3, line 527).

In *The Wanderings of Oisin*, the "unguents out of flowers" share similarities with self-heal (book 2, line 185). Culpeper writes that self-heal was a "herb of Venus" that patients used to heal themselves and adds that "[i]t is a special herb for inward and outward wounds" (170). When it was used to treat the exterior of the body, it was administered as an "unguent" (Culpeper 170). Culpeper claims that self-heal was used "to cleanse the foulness of sores, and cause them more speedily to be healed" (170). Just as with the medicinal effects of vervain in particular, Yeats removed

[31] *NFCS* 0845: 233; James Cullen (c. 60), Smartscastle West, County Kilkenny. Collector: Strang's Mills, Kilmacow (school), Strangsmill, County Kilkenny, January 1938–January 1939. Teacher: Richard Rellis.

non-Irish additions that were toxic to the Revival of Ireland in its fullest sense, whilst also healing international relations.

In *The Countess Cathleen*, healing is associated with a wandering that is seen as weakness at the exposition, yet it becomes a strength at the resolution. Initially, when Cathleen "wandered in the wood," she claims that she "should know [her] way" (sc. 1, lines 78–79). Shortly afterwards, however, Cathleen reveals that the "doctors bid me fly the unlucky times / And find distraction for my thoughts, or else / Pine to my grave," and therefore encourage a wandering and fleeting mind (lines 116–18). In Cathleen's aim to "shelter all that starve or wander," Aleel claims that "we labour in vain," which echoes the Victorian belief that there was no way of valuing and celebrating leisure and time off (sc. 3, lines 473, 488). In response to Aleel's utilitarian comment about arduous work and toil, Cathleen asks "[h]ow would that quiet end?" (line 489). Aleel answers with another interrogative: "How but in healing?" (line 490). Reciprocating Cathleen's comment that Aleel has "seen [her] tears" and that she could "see [his] hand shake on the floor," he replies that he "thought but of healing" (lines 490–92). The devils, embodied by the merchants, speak about healing herbs in a negative sense. Mary, who is married to the peasant Shemus Rua, states that "God is all-powerful" (sc. 2, line 280). In response to this statement, the second merchant says:

> Pray, you shall need Him.
> You shall eat dock and grass, and dandelion,
> Till that low threshold there becomes a wall,
> And when your hands can scarcely drag your body
> We shall be near you. (lines 280–84)

Although the polysyndetic "dock and grass, and dandelion" were intended as a poor alternative to nourishing food, they contain healing properties for certain illnesses. Dock leaves, for example, were used to cure liver problems in so far as "[t]he leaves of plantain, wild sage, the shamrock and dock-leaf, with valerian and the flower of the daisy" were "plucked by the person before sunrise, and fasting, on Mondays and Wednesdays, while Hail Mary is said, and the Paternoster" and then "boiled and strained, and the herbs afterwards to be carefully burned" (Wilde, *Ancient Cures* 37–38). However, folklore collector Minnie Moore gathered an anonymous account for *The Schools' Manuscript Collection* (*NFCS*), which identifies weeds as "harmful herbs" and further identifies "[s]cutch grass and hair grass" as "very bad weeds" as "the people sowed bad grass-seed" ("Herbs" 174).[32] In Patrick Galavan's folklore collection in *The Schools' Manuscript Collection*, informant Bridget Doran notes that "[t]he dandelion cures bad lungs" ("Herb Cures" 92).[33] Wilde records that "a potion made of dandelion (dent-de-lion—lion's tooth)" was used to treat asthma, and dandelion was also incorporated into an old De Danaan porridge remedy:

> A porridge advised by Dianecht, chief physician of the Tuatha-de-Danans, has been handed down through the centuries for relief of ailments of the body, as cold, phlegm, throat cats, and the presence of living things in the body, as worms. It consists of hazel-buds, dandelion, chickweed, and wood sorrel, all boiled together with oatmeal. This porridge to be taken morning and evening, when the cold and the trouble will soon disappear. (22, 40)

In 1892, when he first published *The Countess Cathleen*, the passage about the De Danaan and the "three things" that cannot be cured with medicine were absent (sc. 2, line 166); they first appear in the 1895 edition in *Poems* (*VP* sc. 2, line 166). In Scene Two, when Cathleen confesses that "[t]he famine frets [her]," her foster-mother Oona responds with Celtic mythology:

> I have lived now near ninety winters, child,
> And I have known three things no doctor cures—
> Love, loneliness, and famine—nor found refuge
> Other than growing old and full of sleep.
> See you where Oisin and young Niam ride
> Wrapped in each other's arms, and where the Finians
> Follow their hounds along the fields of tapestry,
> How merry they lived once, yet men died then.
> I'll sing the ballad young bard Kevin sang
> By the great door, the light about his head,
> Where he bid you cast off this cloud of care. (lines 164–75)

[32] *NFCS* 1019: 174. Collector: Minnie Moore, Benbawn (school), Binbane, County Cavan, c. 1937–1939. Teacher: M. Gillespie.

[33] *NFCS* 0847: 92; Bridget Doran (50). Collector: Patrick Galavan, The Rower (B.), Inistioge (school), County Kilkenny, October 1937—20 December 1938. Teacher: Risteárd Ó Cuirrín.

The last four lines of this passage and the spelling of Oisin's and Niamh's names differed when they were first written in 1895 and have been subject to some dissections and rebuilding since. Oisin and Niamh were referred to as "Usheen and young Neave" and the De Danaan race are featured:

> Sit down by me, and I will chaunt the song
> About the Danaan nations in their raths
> That Aleel sang for you by the great door
> Before we lost him in the shadow of leaves. (*Poems* 94)

As the herbal remedies cannot cure "[l]ove, loneliness, and famine," Yeats again turns to Irish mythology as a mode for healing national wounds and a medicine for ailments that do not respond to folk treatments.

* * *

Having a richly stocked memory in which to wander itself had therapeutic power. Yeats subverts the primary definition of "wandering" as travelling "without fixed course or certain aim," and remoulds it as a healthy framework for both finding and retaining the Irish past ("Wandering"; *OED*). The genesis of Yeats's wanderings began on a childhood visit to County Sligo. These wanderings were prompted by his cousin, Lucy Middleton, who told of fairies stealing "the silver mounting on a walking-stick" in "Ballisodare or Rosses," which is recorded in an autobiography that Yeats published in 1916 titled *Reveries Over Childhood and Youth* (*Autobiographies* 88).[34] This, in addition to Yeats's own apparitional sighting of a man with "no human footstep" in Knocknarea, inspired his earliest folklore-collecting forays (89). Far from being futile, even his first wanderings were filled with purpose: "From that on I wandered about raths and faery hills and questioned old women and old men and, when I was tired out or unhappy, began to long for some such end as True Thomas found" (89).[35]

[34] Yeats writes, "Once she had lost her way in a familiar field, and when she found it again the silver mounting on a walking-stick belonging to her brother which she carried had vanished. An old woman in the village said afterwards, 'You have good friends amongst them, and the silver was taken instead of you'" (Yeats, *Autobiographies* 88).

[35] "True Thomas" is a reference to Jesus's apostle, who did not believe the other disciples when they told him about Jesus's resurrection. As described in the Gospel of John, Thomas says, "Unless I see in [H]is hands the print of the nails, and place my finger in the mark of the nails, and place my hand in [H]is side, I will not believe" (*Holy Bible*, John 20.25). When

A richly stocked memory, of a kind that had been furnished by gleanings from many wanderings, was a defence against extremism. As wandering is strength, Yeats heals the forgotten so that remembrance can flourish. He allows his protagonist to suffer so that the Irish wounds are healed "with unguents out of flowers" (book 2, line 185). As evidenced from his medical language in his thirty-third journal entry within *Estrangement*, an autobiography that records his own memories from 1909, Yeats is aware that the human mind can choose to accept and reject information if the past is not properly remedied:

> All empty souls tend to extreme opinion. It is only in those who have built up a rich world of memories and habits of thought that extreme opinions affront the sense of probability. Propositions, for instance, which set all the truth upon one side can only enter rich minds to dislocate and strain, if they can enter at all, and sooner or later the mind expels them by instinct.[36] (*Autobiographies* 347)

Yeats's main Revivalist idea did not aimlessly wander through his work, but it strode with purpose into his writing from the outset. This was the belief that he could heal a dislocated Irish heritage and reposition it into a new form, much like the "dull and unsubduable" demon that morphed into a "new-healed shape" in *The Wanderings of Oisin* (book 2, lines 221). This poem tracks Oisin's development from being an immortal in the Land of Youth (Tír na nÓg) to the last-remaining Fenian in Ireland, hoping to return to them in death either "in flames or at feast" (book 3, 224). In exchange for a mortal body that ages and decays, Oisin brings his mythological memories back to his homeland.

In a letter to the Dublin-born writer Katharine Tynan, dated 6 September 1888, Yeats states that "I have buried my youth and raised over it a cairn—of clouds" on writing *The Wanderings of Oisin* (*Letters to Katharine Tynan* 64). This statement is reminiscent of the cloudy scenes

"Jesus came and stood among" His disciples, He said "[p]eace be with you" to them all and "[t]hen [H]e said to Thomas, 'Put your finger here, and see [M]y hands; and put out your hand, and place it in [M]y side; do not be faithless, but believing'" (20.26–27). Then, "Thomas answered [H]im, 'My Lord and my God!'" and Jesus said that "[y]ou have believed because you have seen [M]e" and "[b]lessed are those who have not seen and yet believe" (20.28–29). By referencing John 20.19–29 in the notes that accompany Yeats's *Reveries Over Childhood and Youth*, editors William H. O'Donnell and Douglas N. Archibald make it clear that Yeats is alluding to Thomas the Apostle (*Autobiographies* 89).

[36] Yeats did not assign a date to this journal entry.

in his epic poem, where the "wandering and milky smoke" obscures the setting (book 3, lines 1, 12, 148). Despite becoming a Revival masterpiece, Yeats initially had doubts about the clarity of *The Wanderings of Oisin and Other Poems* (1889):

> I am not very hopeful about the book. Somewhat inarticulate have I been, I fear. Something I had to say. Don't know that I have said it[.] All seems confused, incoherent, inarticulate. Yet this I know, I am no idle poetaster. My life has been in my poems. To make them I have broken my life in a mortar, as it were. I have brayed in it youth and fellowship, peace and worldly hopes. I have seen others enjoying, while I stood alone with myself—commenting, commenting—a mere dead mirror on which things reflect themselves. I have buried my youth and raised over it a cairn—of clouds. Some day I shall be articulate, perhaps. But this book I have no great hopes of—it is all sluggish, incoherent. It may make a few friends, perhaps, among people of my own sort—that is the most. Do what you can for it. (*Letters to Katharine Tynan* 64)

It seems that Yeats thinks that his wandering has gone too far—into incoherence. His zest for wandering as a form of therapeutic medicine and a literary technique is complicated with the consideration that wandering has its limits, and the realisation that one can wander too much.

* * *

For Yeats, wandering is also rooted in spirituality in both his personal life and fiction. Based on a reception that opened a performance, the journalist William Bulfin described him as "wander[ing] about like a troubled soul in spiritland or elsewhere" and that "[h]e wanders in the realms of the mind, just as he does in the physical world – taking little note of where his steps are leading him" (qtd. in Foster, *Apprentice Mage* 280).[37] Yeats debated "the independent existence of the wandering spirit mind" (Foster, *Arch-Poet* 73). This spiritual affiliation with wandering speaks into his literary work. In "To the Rose upon the Rood of Time" (1893), a poem that apostrophises and personifies a rose, Yeats writes about "[e]ternal beauty

[37] On 24 October 1902, Yeats attended an opening performance reception, held prior to the publication of his revolutionary play *Where There is Nothing* (1902) that was printed in the *United Irishman* on 30 October 1902 (Foster, *Apprentice Mage* 279).

wandering on her way" (*VP* line 12; Larrissy 60).[38] Edward Larrissy proposes that *The Rose* (1893), a collection of mythological poems, demonstrates that "Yeats seeks to provide a syncretic account of the connections between Ireland and the philosophy of wandering through eternity" (59). Larrissy, in his chapter "Husks, Wandering and the Nation," argues that two pastoral poems, "The Madness of King Goll" (1889) and "Ephemera" (1889), make "covert reference to the doctrine of transmigration, the ultimate form of wandering" (59).[39] Yeats did not only restrict wandering to the physical and literary world, but he saw it as a passage to the supernatural realms.

A wandering spirit helps rather than hinders poetry-writing, as Larrissy postulates that "there is a felicitous kind of acceptance of wandering and contrariety which gives rise to [j]oy" and "[t]his acceptance and this [j]oy, it seems reasonable to infer, are the true preconditions for happy poetic making" (36). He contrasts this with "[t]he spirit that, as the Druids saw, wanders through all things" and "must not be fixed," which "was also an important part of Blake's message" (36). The "[e]ternal beauty wandering on her way" in "To the Rose upon the Rood of Time" is testimony to a higher plain of "wandering" that Yeats aims to access through his poetry (60, 65). Wandering is a space that allows the writer to spiritually travel, explore the contraries in both themselves and society as a whole, and record this in the human world on paper.

* * *

The Wanderings of Oisin is an allegory of recovery and revival that links to the medical preoccupations of "wandering." Yeats deploys "wandering" and "wavering" in order to clear the dust away from forgotten Irish texts and halt their decay through transplanting them into a new body of popular culture (book 1, line 275). The line, "[w]e passed by woods, and lawns of clover," is built with iambic tetrameter and sounds like the wandering and walking footsteps of Oisin, placing one foot in front of the other

[38] Larrissy provides an interpretation of this quotation in his chapter, "Rose, Mirror and Hem," in his *Yeats the Poet: The Measures of Difference* (1994) on pages 60–71.

[39] "Ephemera" is a pastoral poem that ponders upon the theme of eternity and includes a dialogue between two characters with "wandering hearts" (line 12). "The Madness of King Goll" is about a mythological king, whose battling causes him "[*m*]*adness*" (81). It is a "whirling and a wandering fire" that "grew" in his "secret spirit" that prompted him to "wander in the woods" without a sense of fulfilment (lines 27–28, 37).

(book 1, line 377). In his first version of *The Wanderings of Oisin*, published in 1889, Yeats adapts this line to: "By woods of moss, by lawns of colours" (book 1, line 377; textual variants). He changes "moss" to "woods" in his second version that was printed in 1895 in *Poems*, when the line reads, "We passed by woods, and lawns of clover" (22). This deletion of moss is perhaps Yeats's way of clearing decay, as moss is a sign of neglect ("Moss"; *OED*). It also has magical and healing properties, which are discussed in the next chapter. In *The Wanderings of Oisin*, the "sea-weed-covered pillars" and "Manannan's dark tower, stone after stone" that "[g]ather[s] sea-slime" are reminiscent of the "sea-green slates" that are built into Thoor Ballylee and the poem "To be Carved on a Stone at Thoor Ballylee" (book 2, lines 32, 236–37; line 2). The anapestic hexameter within the line that reads, "And dwell in the house of the Fenians, be they in flames or at feast," emphasises how Yeats has guided Oisin to bring Irish heritage back home again. Thoor Ballylee was Yeats's own Tír na nÓg, which he built up as a healthy body in which to house Irish literature (book 3, line 224). Yeats's framing to the story is "wandering," and he is reclaiming "wandering" as a positive.

It is important to note that Yeats is perhaps not quite so sanguine about the tower's potential. In the poetry of the twenties and thirties, its "[h]alf dead" condition might be taken as a commentary on a partitioned Ireland, and the potential to "heal" that division was not an option at this stage (line 12; "Blood and the Moon"). Yeats's imagination takes fire from disunity for all his praise of unity of culture and being. "Sailing to Byzantium" (1927), as T. Sturge Moore recognised, ends with the golden bird singing of exactly what the speaker had declared he was leaving—"[t]hat ... country," that is, a disunified Ireland which is "no country for old men" (line 1). In a letter to T. Sturge Moore, written on 7 April 1930, Yeats admits that "I have been ill for five months—Malta Fever, a form of malaria, most of the time—but for some time now have been convalescent and for the last few days have been working every morning a little" (*Correspondence* 160). T. Sturge Moore replies on 16 April 1930:

> I am glad that your worst sufferings are forgotten and that you are now enjoying a luxurious convalescence. Convalescence is always a sort of renewed childhood, with the refreshing discovery of returning powers and the indulgence it wins on all hands.... Your *Sailing to Byzantium*, magnificent as the first three stanzas are, lets me down in the fourth, as such a goldsmith's bird is as much nature as a man's body, especially if it only sings

> like Homer and Shakespeare of what is past or passing or to come to Lords and Ladies. (162)

The poems that immediately follow in *The Tower* (1928) collection all take their inspiration from ruins, disunity, and decay, rather than the unity for which Byzantium seems to be a symbol. The bird, "set upon a golden bough to sing / To lords and ladies of Byzantium / Of what is past, or passing, or to come" is nevertheless a hope that the ailing Irish tradition will invoke a medico-literary response that would generate a greater medical and spiritual healing process for both Ireland and the wider world (lines 30–32).

The Wanderings of Oisin is ultimately an allegory of strength and weakness, and Yeats desires to reassign his work and the Revival from age, illness, and decrepitude to renewed power. The Revival poem's title, layout, content, rhythm, and line lengths are all germane to the theme of "wandering," and both visually and metaphorically demonstrate this ancient and powerful concept. The ethics of the necessity of "wandering" runs throughout this entire epic poem, Yeats's personal life and, by extension, his whole body of writing as a corpus. He was not afraid to chisel out the old in order to carve the Irish Revival into a healthier shape and recapitulate the central theme of preservation. Through *The Wanderings of Oisin* and *The Countess Cathleen*, Yeats gave immunity to his early ideas of Revival. As Yeats's epic poem progresses, the wandering verses grow in length and mirror his walking mind. Due to his meandering thoughts, far from a medical affliction, Irish heritage is no longer wandering around in the past; it has been given a fixed and permanent home in the present and future too. "Wandering" had been seen as a weakness, but Yeats recasts it as a resource and source of strength: a means by which Ireland will regain the flexibility to recover and follow a wandering path to recovery. Several years later, Yeats first wandered the area around Coole-Ballylee, collecting the broken fragments of Irish folklore and building them into a new indigenous body. Reclaiming wandering from a medical sign of weakness to a restorative quality of the spirit was an important part of Yeats's project. It was something that could be brought from the Land of the Young to a debilitated present-day Ireland. He was to find his real-life Tír na nÓg at Thoor Ballylee.

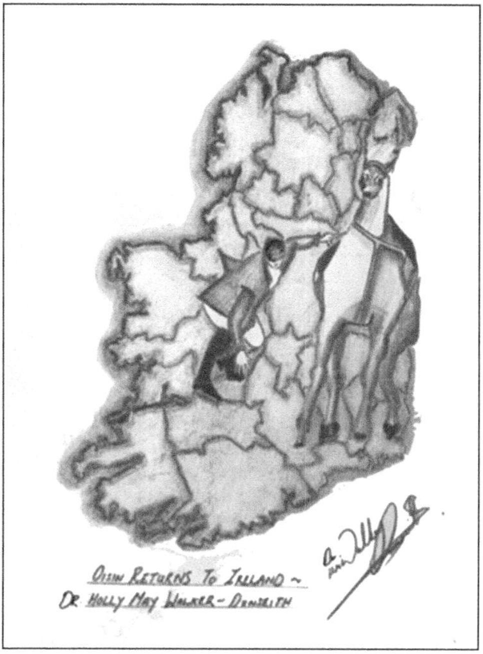

Oisin Returns to Ireland

CHAPTER 3

Thoor Ballylee: Healing and Recovery

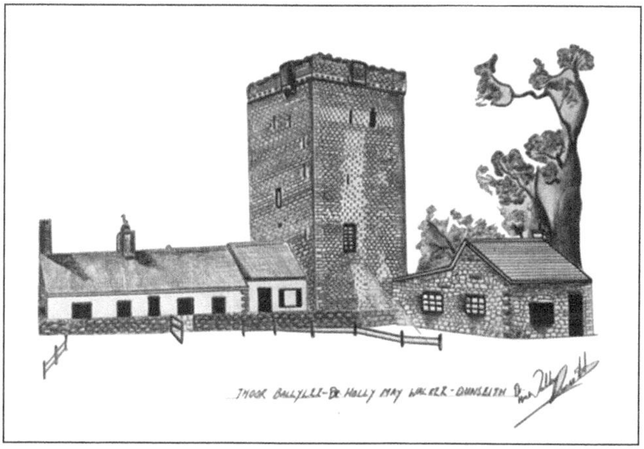

Thoor Ballylee

William Butler Yeats imagined his mediaeval stone tower, which he purchased in 1916, as a living organism. It was "[h]alf dead at the top" and prone to ageing and decay, but its stonework contained crevices that were alive with birds and bees, and it contained the potential for resuscitation,

H. M. Walker-Dunseith, *Traditional Medicine in the Irish Literary Revival*, New Directions in Irish and Irish American Literature,
https://doi.org/10.1007/978-3-031-82459-3_3

restoration, and recovery (line 12; "Blood and the Moon").[1] The restoration of his tower was also a restoration back to health, as Yeats simultaneously recovered his own health after the shocks of the 1916 Rising and the tumultuous circumstances of his marriage in the years after its purchase. At the same time, he was tending to the primary aim of the Irish Literary Revival: to resuscitate and revive to full health an ailing Irish heritage. To Yeats, this meant joining different elements that might grow together: the semi-submerged Irish tradition could knit with the "bloody, arrogant" energies of the "men-at-arms, cross-gartered to the knees," who built the tower, and with the best courtly and intellectual traditions of the Anglo-Irish world as it was represented by great houses like the nearby Coole Park (line 3; "Blood and the Moon"; line 82; "The Tower"). Through healing Thoor Ballylee, by extension, he was repairing a fractured Ireland following the Easter Rising and a wounded world following the First World War. Not only is the tower somewhere that Yeats restored, it is also a place that could, in his imagination, contribute to wider spiritual and societal restoration. Ideas of healing, revival, and recovery were built into the restored walls of Thoor Ballylee itself.

The landscape from which Thoor Ballylee rose had long been associated by Yeats with recovered health. In both 1896 and 1897, Yeats recovered from ill health whilst at Coole Park, which stood nearby. Yeats's first visit to the environs of Thoor Ballylee was in August 1896, and from his

[1] Yeats's "Blood and the Moon" was first published in the *The Winding Stair* collection in 1929, and it is home to his famous statement concerning the property: "I declare this tower is my symbol" (*VP* line 16). "Blood and the Moon" (1929) is a visual poem, as evidenced in Helen Vendler's *Our Secret Discipline: Yeats and Lyric Form* (2007), where she identifies in the shape of the poem on the page an image of the tower itself (81). Vendler writes that "Yeats chooses, in 'Blood and the Moon' (as in no other sequence), a graphic, pictorial method of arrangement" (81). She notes, "In the first 'station' of the sequence he will show us, from the outside, the tall shape of the tower he has restored; then, in the second station (part II) he will laboriously climb its stair, stopping from time to time; and finally, in the third and fourth stations in the upper chamber of the tower (parts III and IV), he will contemplate its windows" (81). She claims, "He is tempted to rise to the upper ruined battlement, but he breaks off before he does so, and the battlement does not generate any pictorial equivalent of itself" (81). This visual poem, which connects Thoor Ballylee to Irish history, was born out of Irish politician and Free State Minister Kevin O'Higgins's assassination in 1927. Yeats remembered his friend as Ireland's own "great builder of a nation" in a sympathetic letter to the widowed Brigid O'Higgins (*Uncollected Prose* 476). On 14 July 1927, this letter was printed in the *Irish Times* newspaper (476). Furthermore, "The Tower" is a bucolic poem within his 1928 collection, wielding the same title. It explores "[d]ecrepit age" in relation to the tower, its builders, and past inhabitants (line 3).

first encounter with the place it is associated with a narrative of recovery from ill health. In "Book V: The Stirring of the Bones" within the autobiography *The Trembling of the Veil* (1922), Yeats admits that he was "in poor health" because "the strain of youth had been greater than it commonly is, even with imaginative men, who must always, I think, find youth bitter" and he "could neither write nor cease to write" his forever unfinished novel—*The Speckled Bird* (*Autobiographies* 282–83).[2] Lady Gregory "drove over to Tulira, and after Symons' return to London [Yeats] stayed at her house" on a day trip, a visit he identifies as marking the start of his recovery (282). On this first stay, he took part in folklore collection in the district with Gregory as an antidote to his illness:

> Lady Gregory, seeing that I was ill, brought me from cottage to cottage to gather folk-belief, tales of the faeries, and the like, and wrote down herself what we had gathered, considering that this work, in which one let others talk, and walked about the fields so much, would lie, to use a country phrase, "very light upon the mind." She asked me to return there the next year, and for years to come I was to spend my summers at her house. When I was in good health again, I found myself indolent, partly perhaps because I was affrighted by that impossible novel, and asked her to send me to my work every day at eleven, and at some other hour to my letters, rating me with idleness if need be, and I doubt if I should have done much with my life but for her firmness and her care. After a time, though not very quickly, I recovered tolerable industry, though it has only been of late years that I have found it possible to face an hour's verse without a preliminary struggle and much putting off. (283)

In his late memoir *Dramatis Personae: 1896–1902* (1935), Yeats again connected his recovery from ill health with the work he did at Coole. He remembered that, when he arrived, his "health was giving way" and his "nerves had been wrecked" (*Autobiographies* 298). He again remembered how, in response to this, Gregory sprung into action: "Finding that I could not work, and thinking the open air salutary, Lady Gregory brought me from cottage to cottage collecting folk-lore" (298).

Yeats returned, as Gregory requested, the following year in 1897, and was again in need of recovery from illness (*Autobiographies* 282–84,

[2] Yeats states that "I had lost myself besides, as I had done periodically for years, upon Hodos Chameliontos" (*Autobiographies* 282).

298–99).[3] In this second recovery, he confessed in *Dramatis Personae* that he had been suffering from lost love and chronic heartbreak (*Autobiographies* 298–99). The cause of this, according to Yeats, was Maud Gonne's repeated refusals of his marriage proposals since 1891. In addition to this, Olivia Shakespear's decision to end her and Yeats's affair contributed to the, in Yeats's words, "disappointed love" that "tortured" him (qtd. in Donoghue, *Memoirs* 125). In his *Memoirs*, Yeats states that "[i]t was a time of great personal strain and sorrow" because "[s]ince [his] mistress [Olivia Shakespear] had left [him], no other woman had come into [his] life, and for nearly seven years none did" (qtd. in Donoghue 125). The keynote of his earliest encounters with Coole Park is the restoration of health, and the Coole-Thoor Ballylee area never lost these associations for him.

The connections between Coole-Ballylee (the latter of which stands on grounds that formerly belonged to the Coole estate) and restored health run very deep in his imagination and writing. The alliance between Coole-Ballylee and recovered mental health is attested to in the title poem to *In the Seven Woods* (1904), a poem that begins ominously:

> I have heard the pigeons of the Seven Woods
> Make their faint thunder, and the garden bees
> Hum in the lime-tree flowers; … (lines 1–3)

[3] Information about Yeats's recovery from illness can be found in "Book V. The Stirring of the Bones" within *The Trembling of the Veil*, and it can also be seen in *Dramatis Personae*. I have found two instances of recovery in association with Coole Park and Lady Gregory's folklore-collecting forays. The initial recovery appears to occur on Yeats's first visit to Coole Park in 1896, when Lady Gregory "whom [Yeats] had met once in London for a few minutes, drove over to Tulira, and after Symons' return to London [Yeats] stayed at her house" (*Autobiographies* 282; "The Stirring of the Bones"). He was emotionally wounded from "the strain of youth," alongside encountering obstacles with his unfinished novel—*The Speckled Bird* (282). Yeats's next recovery happens on his second visit to Coole Park the following summer in 1897. This is when he suffers from his recent separation from Olivia Shakespear, and Maud Gonne's more long-term rejection of his marriage proposals due to unrequited love. Gregory treats both examples of illness in the same way. In both 1896 and 1897, she nurses Yeats back to health by bringing him on folklore-collecting forays in the hope that this would be therapeutic. This revival of Yeats's health, brought about by natural lifestyle changes, is a stark contrast to his approach to recovery in 1934. Following Gregory's death on 22 May 1932, and therefore the loss of a strong support system, Yeats turned to medicine rather than therapeutics. This took the form of his rejuvenation through the Steinach Operation, which Yeats underwent two years later on either 5 or 6 April 1934, almost in exactly the same month as Gregory's passing.

These healing bees "put away / The unavailing outcries and the old bitterness / That empty the heart" and pave the way for the personified "Quiet" that "[w]anders laughing and eating her wild heart / Among pigeons and bees" (lines 10–12). In both his personal life and literary works, Coole and Ballylee are united with nature, recovery, and the medicinal bees that replenish and refresh both the natural environment and the worldly tensions that affect it.

It is perhaps significant that Yeats recalled how Gregory sought to restore his strength through bringing him on folklore-collecting forays, as this practice itself sought to revive the subdued Irish energies that, in her eyes and those of other Revivalists, were falling prey to the encroachments of modernity. For Yeats, a personal narrative of the recovery of health, and a national narrative of the recovery of the Irish past, supported by the order and rigour of Coole Park, were linked. These ideas were to have a profound effect on how he was to eventually view the nearby tower that he bought in 1916.

As always, on the contrary, Yeats's visions of unity and healing are in a dialectical relationship with disunity and destruction. It is telling that "the tower" is the tarot card which, blasted by lightning, has a dual connotation: destruction and the flash or bolt of inspiration (line 47). The tower tarot card is a deeply disturbing major arcana card that, among its many catastrophic and destructive implications, can indicate illness and be connected to spiritual sickness and physical disease. Yeats would have been well aware of this meaning. Edward Larrissy proposes that "Yeats became once again a spokesman for his nation, and might be said at last to have forged for it an image of unity" although "this was a development that had to wait for a few years" (*Yeats the Poet* 179). He notes that "a broad reaction against 'bitterness,' ... is bound up with 'brokenness'" (179). Larrissy claims that "[a]t a more general level," Yeats "associates violence and bitterness with the antithetical and demonic," which is exacerbated by "the [t]arot pack, with which, as a member of the Golden Dawn, he had acquired a deep familiarity" (165). "The [t]ower" is also a "[t]arot trump card" that "shows a tower with its top struck off by a zig-zag of lightning," which of course resonates with Yeats's own tower that is "[h]alf dead at the top" (Larrissy 165; *VP* line 12). Furthermore, Larrissy writes that "Kathleen Raine points out that initiates would have associated this image with the downward path of inspiration" (165; Raine 238–44). Larrissy adds that "[t]he normal path of the initiate was to toil upwards through the spheres of the [t]ree of [l]ife; but God descending through the [t]ree was the unasked inspiration" (165). There is still hope for a spiritual healing due to Jesus Christ's ultimate sacrifice for the world's sin. Although Yeats's tower—like the fallen world—was broken, there is still chance for healing and salvation through an amalgamation of different elements that might grow together regardless of their brokenness.

The tower itself represents healing and recovery. It is an amalgam of fragments from the Irish past, and it is a microcosm of various contradictions in Ireland that are melded into a unity. The Anglo-Normans invaded Ireland in the twelfth century, and they became the original authors of Yeats's tower, which was constructed at some point between the fourteenth and sixteenth centuries (Yeats, inevitably, preferred an earlier date).[4] Though the arrival of powerful Norman clans like the de Burgos, who built the tower, is more often associated with ideas of conquest and the assertion of power, and thus Ireland's history of violence and colonisation, there are other elements that are visible in the environs of Ballylee as well. The thatched cottage that adjoins the stone tower connects it to the vernacular architecture of the locality and that of the wider Irish countryside. Furthermore, the millboards that Yeats used in the tower's restoration link the building to a local myth of healing, and to the practitioner Biddy Early.

* * *

[4] Although the sixteenth century was not "Norman," Yeats nevertheless describes his Thoor Ballylee as a Norman tower. In a letter to Herbert Edward Palmer, a literary critic and poet, Yeats writes: "I live in a mediaeval Tower in the West of Ireland" (qtd. in Wade 689). In the second part of "Meditations in Time of Civil War" (1928), labelled "My House," Yeats refers to "[a]n ancient bridge, and a more ancient tower" (line 1). He also mentions the "Norman upland" in "Owen Aherne and his Dancers" in 1928 (line 2). Both of these poems are situated in the 1928 collection, aptly titled *The Tower*. In *The Arch-Poet*, R. F. Foster notes Yeats's statement, directed towards doctor (otolaryngologist) and poet Oliver St. John Gogarty, that was written in a diary belonging to literary scholar Horace M. Reynolds: "The Normans had form, Gogarty, the Normans had form" (qtd. in Foster 84; Reynolds b Ms Am 1787 [5803]). In "To be Carved on a Stone at Thoor Ballylee," belonging to the *Michael Robartes and the Dancer* (1921) collection, Yeats claims that he "restored this tower" using "old mill boards and sea-green slates" (line 2). In October 1916, Yeats inquired about purchasing the Ballylee Castle, and he negotiated the land and cost in November; on 19 November, he visited the property, accompanied by a builder (Foster, *Arch-Poet* 84). Foster writes that "[o]n 27 March [1917] he accepted it for £35" and "on 30 June 1917, WBY [William Butler Yeats] signed the deed of sale" (85).

Among the folklore that Yeats learned on his forays around Coole Park were stories of the folk healer Biddy Early, a figure who plays an intriguing role in Yeats's earliest encounter with the tower. She was a County Clare wise woman, credited with magical healing abilities. Folklore sources show that she was often associated with the fairies because it was believed that she could predict the future and heal illnesses using herbs and a magic bottle (Burke 3).[5] Yeats records discussing her in a conversation with a Ballylee miller in 1896, when he was visiting his theatrical collaborator Edward Martyn at nearby Tulira Castle. Yeats's earliest encounter with the tower at Ballylee in 1896, which he would later christen as "Thoor Ballylee," was also an encounter with Early.[6]

> I HAVE been lately to a little group of houses, not many enough to be called a village, in the barony of Kiltartan in County Galway, whose name, Ballylee, is known through all the west of Ireland. There is the old square castle, Ballylee, inhabited by a farmer and his wife, and a cottage where their daughter and their son-in-law live, and a little mill with an old miller, and old ash-trees throwing green shadows upon a little river and great stepping stones. I went there two or three times last year to talk to the miller about Biddy Early, a wise woman that lived in Clare some years ago, and about her saying, "There is a cure for all evil between the two mill-wheels of Ballylee,"

[5] John Rainsford states that "[t]he first account of Biddy Early's life appeared in 1903" ("Biddy Early's Limerick Connections" 45). This takes the form of journalist R. Burke's "The Last of the Irish Witches," a newspaper article published on 10 October 1903 in the *Weekly Irish Times* (3). This "was followed by Lady Isabella Augusta Gregory's 'Visions and Beliefs in the West of Ireland' (1920)" (Rainsford 45). Richard Jenkins proposes that "[a] piece in *The Limerick Chronicle* on 29 July 1869, reporting her fourth marriage, may be Biddy Early's first appearance in print" (167). In this article, Early is portrayed as "an old woman known as 'Biddy Early' who resides near Tulla, and who, among the peasantry, has the reputation of a witch or sorceress, who could cure all kinds of diseases" (qtd. in Jenkins 167; qtd. in Ryan 87). However, it is more likely that Early's name was first printed on 28 September 1853 in *The Limerick Chronicle*, where she was termed "a fairy doctoress" ("House Burning"). This article records that Tom Flannery, Early's third husband, was accused of deliberately burning down a house.

[6] Yeats reveals his chosen name for the tower, which he christens as "Thoor Ballylee," in his letter to Olivia Shakespear (composed in April 1922): "What do you think of our address—Thoor Ballylee? Thoor is Irish for tower and it will keep people from suspecting us of modern gothic and a deer park. I think the harsh sound of 'Thoor' amends the softness of the rest" (qtd. in Wade, *Letters* 680). Years before this, on 23 July 1918, Yeats uses a heading in a letter to art and manuscript collector John Quinn, which reads as "*Ballylee Castle*[,] *Gort, Co. Galway*" and he confides that "[t]his heading is written in hope, that is to say, I hope it will be true a day or two after this letter reaches you, at the latest" (qtd. in *Letters* 651).

> and to find out from him or another whether she meant the moss between the running waters or some other herb. I have been there this summer, and I shall be there again before it is autumn, because Mary Hynes, a beautiful woman whose name is still a wonder by turf fires, died there sixty years ago; for our feet would linger where beauty has lived its life of sorrow to make us understand that it is not of the world. (Yeats, *Mythologies* 14)

Just as Early's patients actively travelled to her abode in order to seek her medical help, Yeats similarly sought out the miller who possessed information regarding the cure that Early commented upon—the healing "moss ... or some other herb." It is probable that this curiosity about recovery was influenced by Yeats's own desired recuperation from illness and heartbreak at the time. The conversation connecting Early and Ballylee is recorded in "Dust Hath Closed Helen's Eyes" (1899). In *Thoor Ballylee—Home of William Butler Yeats*, Mary Hanley and Liam Miller note that this essay was previously published in the less substantial version of *The Celtic Twilight* in 1893, and in the October 1899 edition of the aestheticist arts periodical *The Dome* (12). Eventually published in Yeats's *The Celtic Twilight* (1902), his encounter with the miller forms the crux of Early's link to Thoor Ballylee. Just as ligaments join bone to bone, Early is the connective tissue that links the folkloric, the occult, and medicine. This raises an interesting question about the role of Early in Yeats's thinking and his rebuilding of the tower, and why he is invested in her healing abilities and so intent to build her into Thoor Ballylee using the millboards.

In addition to his repeated returns to the mill, Yeats's written references to Ballylee indicate how strongly it is associated in his mind with the idea that it is the source of a panacea. This is indicated in his additions to a poem written by his friend AE (born George William Russell), "The Well of All-Healing," which show that ideas of both illness and recovery were turning in the millwheels of his mind[7]:

AE had originally written that "[t]here's a cure for all things in the well at Ballykeele" in his poem that was reprinted within the 1897 periodical, *A Celtic Christmas* (see Fig. 3.1). As a collector, Lady Gregory owned a copy of this publication. Yeats, evidently a tireless reviser of the work of others as well as his own, set to work on this poem, redrafting it according

[7]Yeats refers to "the mill of the mind" in "An Acre of Grass" (1938), a poem about the declining "strength of body" (419) and the pledge that "[m]yself must I remake" (lines 10, 4, 14). Whilst the "acre of green grass / For air and exercise" remains, Yeats has "[an] old man's eagle mind" that becomes "[f]orgotten else by mankind" (lines 2–3, 23–24).

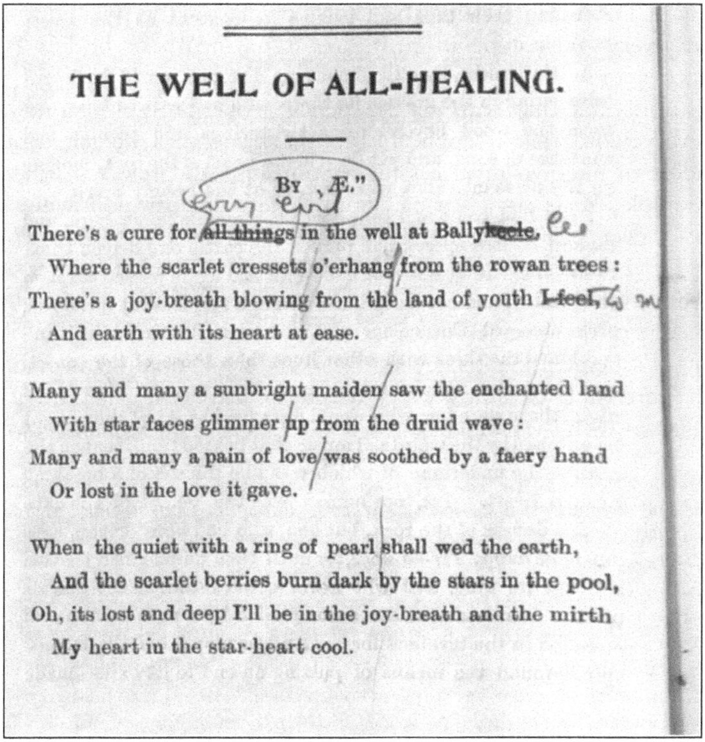
THE WELL OF ALL-HEALING.

By "Æ."

There's a cure for all things in the well at Ballykeele,
Where the scarlet cressets o'erhang from the rowan trees:
There's a joy-breath blowing from the land of youth I feel,
And earth with its heart at ease.

Many and many a sunbright maiden saw the enchanted land
With star faces glimmer up from the druid wave:
Many and many a pain of love was soothed by a faery hand
Or lost in the love it gave.

When the quiet with a ring of pearl shall wed the earth,
And the scarlet berries burn dark by the stars in the pool,
Oh, its lost and deep I'll be in the joy-breath and the mirth
My heart in the star-heart cool.

Fig. 3.1 Yeats's adaptations to AE's "The Well of All-Healing," which is a poem that was republished in *A Celtic Christmas* in 1897. Yeats made his own pencil annotations to this poem within the periodical. Lady Gregory owned this copy, which Yeats would turn into a manuscript revision. The John J. Burns Library at Boston College provided the above image

to his own tastes. In the first line, Yeats crosses out "all things," and replaces it with the alliterative "every evil" (see Fig. 3.1). This change, of course, aligns the poem with the tale told by the miller at Ballylee to whom Yeats had spoken.

This redraft is thought to be where Yeats first wrote down the proper noun "Ballylee" on paper (Pethica, "'Uttering, Mastering it'?" 219). He also changes the third line from "[t]here's a joy-breath blowing from the land of youth I feel" to "[t]here's a joy-breath blowing from the land of youth to me," fatefully yoking together "Ballylee" and "me" in rhyme (see Fig. 3.1).[8] It is interesting that Yeats operates on this poem during his own recovery and recuperation; it is as if a sympathetic healing is taking place.

It is noticeable that Yeats places a pencil stroke, prompting a new line, near every word that is applicable to the heartbreak he felt in 1897, reminders of his own unsuccessful relationships and rejected proposals. For example, Yeats signals a paragraph break after the following word groups: "every evil," "sunbright maiden" and "pain of love" (see Fig. 3.1).[9] He breaks the poem in order to put it back together again, deconstructing the interweaving *ABAB* rhyme scheme and quickening the hexameters of the original into a loose trimeter. Although he demolishes the rhyme scheme using his new line markers, thus bringing dissonance to the first three lines of almost every stanza, he leaves the final line of each stanza intact with the original three-or-so stresses. His freehand rewriting

[8] The "land of youth" is an allusion to *The Lay of Oisín in the Land of Youth*, where health does not diminish and age does not progress. See Micheál Coimín's *Laoi Oisín ar Tír na n-Óg: The Lay of Oisín in the Land of Youth* (1896).

[9] In AE's second line that reads, "Where the scarlet cressets o'erhang from the rowan trees," Yeats's pencil marking is placed after the active verb "o'erhang" (see Fig. 3.1). However, it looks like Yeats originally drew the line after the plural concrete noun "cressets," but then erased this marking, judging from its faint yet present appearance on the page. A "cresset," historically, is defined as "[a] vessel of iron or the like, made to hold grease or oil, or an iron basket to hold pitched rope, wood, or coal, to be burnt for light; usually mounted on the top of a pole or building, or suspended from a roof" ("Cresset"; *OED*). Its now obsolete meaning is "a cavity in a cresset-stone," which is "a flat stone with cup-shaped hollows for holding grease to be burnt for light" ("Cresset"; *OED*). This is interesting because this cresset as cavity is reminiscent of the gap in the house wall that features in Yeats's "The Stare's Nest by My Window" within *The Tower* collection (1928). The cresset as stone that is used for burning light is linked to buildings in so far as it is usually positioned at the summit of a property; perhaps the light is a symbol of hope and health for Yeats. Instead of leaving his pencil marking beside "cresset," he appears to erase this and re-establish the line next to the active verb "o'erhang." As a noun, "o'erhang" is "a projecting part, esp. of rocks or a building"; as a verb, it means "to loom over, overshadow; to threaten" in a figurative sense ("Overhang"; *OED*). Although "o'erhang" perhaps seems a more negative word than "cressets," it could arguably hold positive connotations for Yeats. Rather than looking at the health that is currently missing from his life (symbolised by the cresset as cavity), Yeats is instead looking at the material in his life that is present and in abundance (as symbolised by the verb "o'erhang" that is linked to buildings). This material includes his literary work and folklore-collecting practice, and his future project as restorer of Thoor Ballylee. Both words—the concrete noun "cresset" and active verb "o'erhang"—relate to buildings. Yeats's decision to move the pencil line forwards is perhaps his way of literally drawing a line under his misery and ill health; a way to move forward and leave illness behind.

of AE's poem echoes the willingness to remake and restore that he was to eventually bring to the tower in Ballylee, the one proper name he wrote into the poem. This also repeats the remaking and restoration of the famous lyric "Down by the Salley Gardens" (1889), which, of course, is the product of folklore-collecting and the repair and "reconstruct[ion]" of the fragments of the poem that the "old peasant woman" is able to remember (Yeats, *VP* 90; Yeats's footnote). In a letter to Katharine Tynan on 22–28 September 1888, Yeats writes that "I enclose a couple of lyrics of my own for your opinion" and "[o]ne is made out of three lines of verse I picked up in Sligo—old Irish verse" (*CL* 1: 97). Katharine Tynan mentions in her biographical *The Middle Years* (1893) that the poems that Yeats was referring to in his letter were both "An Isle in the Water" and "Down by the Salley Gardens" (46). John Kelly and Eric Domville, editors for the Oxford collection of Yeats's letters, add that "Down by the Salley Gardens" was "based on the Sligo ballad 'Going to Mass last Sunday my True Love passed me by,'" which "was originally titled 'An Old Song Re-Sung'" (*CL* 1: 97). Yeats did not only renovate buildings, but he also pieced together this old Irish ballad and footnoted that it was "an attempt to reconstruct an old song from three lines imperfectly remembered by an old peasant woman in the village of Ballysodare, Sligo, who often sings them to herself" (qtd. in Kelly and Domville, *CL* 1: 97). This replicates Yeats's mission for both his tower and the world's wounds. The line that reads, "She bid me take life easy, as the grass grows on the weirs," again signifies a rebuilding as a "weir" is a man-made "barrier or dam to restrain water, *esp.* one placed across a river or canal in order to raise or divert the water for driving a mill-wheel" (line 7; "Weir"; *OED*). This weir, applied to waterways "to retain the water and regulate its flow," is prophetic for Yeats's later rebuilding of his tower ("Weir"; *OED*). Although written many years before Yeats purchased the tower in 1916, this line from "Down by the Salley Gardens" still speaks to the human process of rebuilding. Yeats is exercising the wisdom that one must "take life easy" whilst "the grass grows on the weirs," or, in other words, look after one's health as other aspects of life are being rebuilt and falling into place.

In AE's poem, "joy-breath" emanates "from the land of youth"; Lady Gregory advised that the "open air" would be "salutary" for Yeats's recovery (see Fig. 3.1; Yeats, *Autobiographies* 298; *Dramatis Personae*). These words are, in their own ways, reflections of nineteenth-century nostrums that placed the highest value on fresh air and ventilation as both preventatives and cures for illness. Miasmas, it was believed, built up in poorly ventilated spaces and caused illness. To read of oxygenation is to read of the necessary precondition of recovery to the Victorian mind. Already, from his earliest visits to the district in 1896 and 1897, the environs of Coole Park and Ballylee were associated in Yeats's imagination with healing. The miasmatic hypothesis was believed to be the leading aetiology for illness until 1890, when germ theory took centre stage.[10] Meaning "stain" and "defilement" in ancient Greek, miasmas were thought to be a build-up of "[n]oxious vapour" ("Miasma"; *OED*). As an escape from this, Victorian people would visit the seaside or country areas, especially if they had chest complaints.[11] When the sickness-prone Yeats altered AE's poem to link Ballylee and a "joy-breath blowing from the land of youth to me," he was reflecting contemporary medical ideas.

* * *

Biddy Early, whom Yeats associated with the millwheels of Ballylee, joins the concepts of the occult, witchcraft, and healing in Yeats's late memoir, *Dramatis Personae* (*Autobiographies* 299). Written at a time when health concerns were very much on the poet's mind, Yeats recalls a conversation with an elderly shepherd in Doneraile, a town in north County Cork, in which he asks about Early and receives an answer that both deflects him and feeds his interest. Yeats asked:

> "Has anybody ever gone from here to consult Biddy Early?"—a famous Clare witch—and in a moment the man's face became excited; he himself had stood at the roadside, watching spirits playing hurley in a field, until one came and pulled the cap over his eyes. What he saw, what he did not see but thought he saw, does not concern me here, being but a part of that traditional experience which I have discussed only too much elsewhere. That experience is my obsession, as Coole and its history, her hope that her son or her grandson might live there, were Lady Gregory's. (299)

[10] Germ theory gradually overtook miasmatic theory as the reason for disease that manifests in the body. Scientists, such as Louis Pasteur and Robert Koch, progressed this microbe hypothesis so that it became more widely accepted by 1890.

[11] James Johnson, a nineteenth-century royal surgeon, provides a Victorian perspective about the effect of sea air and the climate on both mind and body in his *Change of Air; or, the Diary of a Philosopher in Pursuit of Health and Recreation* (1831) on page 298.

Early, as Yeats's talisman for healing in the west of Ireland, is the spirit of the region. She represents medicine, but also a distinct otherworld that crosses over into the everyday world and thus forms a connection between the two. He evokes the same restorative powers in the introductory rhymes to "The Shadowy Waters" (1900), a dramatic poem in which the sea god Forgael follows souls that are embodied as birds, as "*I walked among the seven woods of Coole*" which "[*w*]*ise Biddy Early called the wicked wood*" (lines 1, 15). Yeats treats the mystical experience of the fairy realm and everyday Irish country life as one and the same. The fact that his question about the earthly Biddy Early prompts an answer about an encounter with fairies is what is significant. Yeats is not entangling himself in a debate about whether fairies are real or not; the experience of hearing the real and the otherworldly bound up without distinction is what fascinates him. For Yeats, this kind of free interchange between this world and others is a sign that contemporary rifts—between ancient and the new, between mystical and scientific worldviews, between Gaeldom and Ireland's other cultures—might be healed.

Early, though, was not represented by Yeats in an entirely positive light. In *The Pot of Broth* (1904), a play exploring the dichotomy between rich and poor, a tramp possesses a magical stone that conjures food. *The Pot of Broth* is a collaborative work of Yeats and Gregory. Its powers are described in his conversation with John and the miserly Sibby Coneely, a married couple who inhabit the cottage kitchen that the tramp trespasses upon. This homeless character recalls an encounter with a mystical "little old man" in a "hareskin coat," who gives him the stone as an exchange: "'Call off your dog,' says he, 'and I'll give you that stone, and if ever you want a good drop of broth or a bit of stirabout, or a drop of poteen itself, all you have to do is to put it down in a pot with a drop of water and stir it awhile, and you'll have the thing you were wanting ready before you'" (lines 178–79, 183, 193–98; act 1). The tramp adds that meat cannot be combined with the broth on Fridays, when Catholics fast, as this would result in a "fistful of bog mould" (line 230). As the stone "has enchantment on it" and can be mixed in a pot with "a bit of an herb for fear the enchantment might slip away from it," such as "[s]lanlus" that is "cut with a black-handed knife" or "a sprig of the [a]thair-talav, the father of herbs" or "leaves" of "*cabbage and onions*," it is an unyielding source of food and prevents hunger (lines 148, 157–61, 166–67, 171). In the Great Famine (1845–1852), approximately one million people—and more—died from hunger as their bodies were denied sustenance and nourishment (Ó Gráda,

Great Irish Famine 1). *The Pot of Broth* strikes a chord with Irish audiences because of the continued presence of memories of this time on the popular psyche at the time Yeats was writing.

Yeats introduces a reference to Early at the resolution, but she is portrayed in a negative light. The parsimonious and credulous Sibby, who has "no more pity in her heart than there's a soul in a dog," is the medium through which Yeats delivers his message (line 52–53). Alongside the paralinguistic feature of "*looking at the stone in her hand*," she exclaims: "Broth of the best, stirabout, poteen, wine itself, he said! And the people that will be coming to see the miracle! I'll be as rich as Biddy Early before I die!" (lines 343–46). Yeats inherited this negative view from Gregory, whose attitudes to Early we can read about in the "Seers and Healers" chapter, a treasury of local accounts about Early, within her larger folklore collection titled *Visions and Beliefs in the West of Ireland* (1920). After Early's death, a mother and daughter resided in her cottage, located "*between Feakle and Tulla*" in County Clare (1: 35). On questioning them, Gregory found out that she was not the only visitor to this healing house. The mother often had to send people away, "*telling them Biddy Early was dead*" (1: 37). Most likely as a joke, a priest advised the mother that "she had a right to shake a bottle and say she was her, and get something from them" (1: 46). Gregory records that this "*friendly priest*," probably in jest, asks, "*Why didn't you let on you were her and make something out of them?*" (1: 37). Another informant of Gregory's, Mrs. Kearns, averred that "her fingers" were "all covered with big gold rings" (1: 40). Mr. McCabe, a past patient of Early's, tells Gregory about the material profits that she allegedly gained from healing:

> There were side-cars and common cars and gentry and country people at the door, just like Gort market, and dinner for all that came, and everyone would bring her something, but she didn't care what it was. Rich farmers would bring her the whole side of a pig. Myself, I brought a bottle of whiskey and a shilling's worth of bread, and a quarter of sugar and a quarter pound of tea. She was very rich, for there wasn't a farmer but would give her the grass of a couple of bullocks or a filly. She had the full of a field of fillies if they'd all been gathered together. (1: 42–43)

If Early's motives were suspected by Gregory and subsequently Yeats, she had many defenders. Leah Butler, writing for the *Women's Museum of Ireland*, blames both a witchcraft trial in 1865 and the Catholic Church for blackening her name ("Biddy Early"). Early was accused of being a witch, and her trial took place in Ennis; she was exculpated due to withdrawn testimonies and support from the peasantry (Butler, "Biddy Early"). Following the Catholic Emancipation in 1829, the Church's scepticism about non-orthodox invocation became a witch-hunt that aimed to eradicate heretics. Michael Hogan (1832–1899), a Limerick-born poet and contemporary of Early's, sought to defend her from the allegations of profiteering that Yeats's play hints at: "She was not a mercenary imposter, for she'd take nothing, neither money nor value, from any person whom she could not serve, and if the required service could be rendered she'd accept nothing but the merest trifle, never surpassing a shilling" (Hogan 267; qtd. in Jenkins 167).[12] This was far from what Gregory had discovered in her investigations, and Early's memory had come down to Yeats with some suspicions of mercenary conduct. He clearly was in two minds about her: if he included a negative comment about her in *The Pot of Broth*, he put this comment in the mouth of an ungenerous, self-centred, and comical character that readers are not likely to take seriously. And, of course, he returned to ask about her several times at the mill she frequented at Ballylee.

Unlike Yeats's character, Sibby, Early is reported to have been "kind" and "willing" (*Visions and Beliefs* 1: 45). Bartley Coen, one of Gregory's informants, insists that "she wasn't *away* herself" but "it was from a son of her own she got the knowledge" (1: 44). On his deathbed, the boy told Early that "the soup of the hen" could heal him (1: 45). Although she succeeded in bringing this soup to him, the boy tells her that "[i]t can't cure me … for no earthly thing can do that" (1: 45). As he saw that she was "kind and willing" and "did her best for [him]," he promised to "leave [her] a way of living" and therefore "taught her all she knew" (1: 45).[13] The source of Early's power has long been in dispute; it has been

[12] Michael Hogan wrote *The Lays and Legends of Thomond* (1880).

[13] James Meaney informs collector Mary O'Loughlin that Early's son "appeared to her after his death" and "told her to look into the bottle before she gave a cure to anyone" ("Biddy Early"; *NFCS* 0596: 126; James Meaney, Creevagh More, County Clare. Collector: Mary O'Loughlin, An Daingean, Cuinche (school), Dangan, County Clare, 1 April 1938–30 June 1938. Teachers: Stiofán Mac Clúin and Treasa Ní Chonmara). This is supported by one of Gregory's informants, Mr. Fahy, who claims that "[a]fter his death always lamenting for him she was, till he came back, and gave her the gift of curing" (*Visions and Beliefs* 45).

attributed to her mother, brother, son and, of course, the fairies.[14] Nevertheless, her "charity and kindness and healing"—as reported by Mr. McCabe—did not go unnoticed, and her reputation in the vicinity when Yeats visited Coole seemed to be an ambiguous one (1: 42).

Yeats was very curious to know whether the cure that he had heard about referred to "the moss between the running waters or some other herb" (*Mythologies* 14). Lady Gregory provides the most likely answer to Yeats's question in her *Visions and Beliefs*. In "Seers and Healers," she writes about Early and the healing moss:

> Biddy Early's cure that you heard of, it was the moss on the water of the mill-stream between the two wheels of Ballylee. It can cure all things brought about by *them* [i.e., fairies], but not any common ailment. But there is no cure for the stroke given by a queen or a fool. There is a queen

[14] The "*Spinning-Woman*" tells Gregory that "Biddy Early was a witch, wherever she got it" (*Visions and Beliefs* 51). Butler, in her article "Biddy Early: The Wise Women of the West," postulates that Early's mother, Ellen Connors (formerly Ellen Early), "had passed on her knowledge of herbal medicine to Biddy" before she died. Based on the information gathered from the "Little Girl of Biddy Early's House," Gregory writes that "[i]t was from her brother that she got the power, when she had to go to the workhouse, and he came back, and gave her the way of doing the cures" (*Visions and Beliefs* 47). Past patient Mr. McCabe, however, asserts that "there's no doubt at all that the reason of her being able to do cures was that she was *away* seven years" (43). He knew this because "[s]he didn't tell [him] about it but she spoke of it to others" (43). The elderly Mr. Saggarton said to Gregory: "Biddy Early told me herself that where she got it was when she was a servant girl in a house, there was a baby lying in the cradle, and he went on living for a few years. But he was friendly to her and used to play tunes for her and when he went away he gave her the bottle and the power. She had but to look in it and she'd see all that had happened and all that was going to happen. But he made her make a promise never to take more than a shilling for any cure she did, and she would not have taken fifty pounds if you offered it to her, though she might take presents of bread and wine and such things" (97). Mrs. Henry, informant in Bernard Regan's collection within *The Schools' Manuscript Collection*, corroborates that "that is how Biddy Early got her charms and that they were all in the bottle," adding that "there was a cure for any disease in the bottle" ("How Biddy Early Got Her Charms"; *NFCS* 0050: 157; Mrs. Henry, grandparent, Gorteenboy, County Galway. Collector: Bernard Regan, Réidh Reamhar (school), Reyrawer, County Galway, c. 1937–1939. Teacher: Seán A. Mac Fhloinn). In Prionnsias Mac Giolla Phóil's collection in *The Schools' Manuscript Collection*, Mrs. John Powell further adds that Early's son (Shawn) won the magic bottle in a hurling match against the fairies ("Biddy Early"; *NFCS* 0591: 272; Mrs. John Powell, collector's mother, parent, Kilbarron, County Clare. Collector: Prionnsias Mac Giolla Phóil, Anach Néill (school), Annaghneal, County Clare, 11 January 1939–31 January 1938. Teacher: B. B. Uí Dhonnchadha).

> in every house or regiment of them. It is of those they steal away they make queens for as long as they live or that they are satisfied with them. (1: 99)

Moss was not efficacious against a queen of fairies, which was a stolen child. This forges a connection with Yeats's early work "The Stolen Child" (1889), which itself has been linked to widespread infant death, including in his own family. The poem is set in his childhood home, County Sligo. The refrain begins with an imperative:

> *Come away, O human child!*
> *To the waters and the wild*
> *With a faery, hand in hand,*
> *For the world's more full of weeping than you can understand.* (lines 24–27)

Two of his older siblings, Robert Corbet and Jane Grace, died early on in their infancy. Roy Foster, Yeats's biographer, confirms that Jane "was born on 29 August 1875, but died less than a year later of bronchial pneumonia," and that Robert was born on 27 March 1870 but "also died in childhood, of croup, at Merville on 3 March 1873" (*Apprentice Mage* 13). Yeats's mother, Susan (née Pollexfen), suffered from depression and was often concerned about her health.[15] For Yeats, "The Stolen Child" carried personal associations as early death was both a societal and individual issue, which may have made tales of the healing moss, and what it could and could not cure, all the more interesting to him.

[15] John and Susan Yeats shared a difficult marriage that was confronted with disagreements, personality differences, financial problems, health concerns, and child death. Alternatively, the Pollexfen family were "apparently rich," and their "milling and shipping interests had prospered and expanded," although neither Susan nor her sisters had access to this fortune (Foster, *Apprentice Mage* 9). Foster describes Susan as "withdrawn and resentful," and he writes that John Butler Yeats "stressed her hatred of his relentless sociability with like-minded artistic and literary friends" (11). Foster notes that John's "letters to her convey exasperation at her anxiety, and her health worries" (11). In a letter dated on 10 November 1872, in response to a concern about weight, John Butler Yeats writes: "I don't know in the least whether it was good or bad—as I don't know what your weight was when last weighed" (qtd. in Foster 12; copies by Susan Mary Yeats/Lily Yeats, NLI MS 2064). Dated 6 February 1873, he observes that "[a]ll your family's ailments begin in the mind a sort of nightmare takes possession of them and they lose their appetite and get ill" (qtd. in Foster 12; copies by Susan Mary Yeats/Lily Yeats, NLI MS 2064). This is reminiscent of Yeats's response to heartbreak, when his "health was giving way" and his "nerves had been wrecked," which needed another visit to Coole in 1897 in order for him to recover (*Autobiographies* 298–99; *Dramatis Personae*).

Gregory cements the links between Coole-Ballylee, Early and the special moss. The Spinning-Woman, an informant, discloses that Early herself "told me she slept in Ballylee mill last night, and that there was a cure for all things in the world between the two wheels there" (*Visions and Beliefs* 1: 52). This local interviewee, in conversation with Gregory, explores the possible reasons behind Early's knowledge of both the mill's whereabouts and the cure itself: "And she said there was a cure for all sicknesses hidden between the two wheels of Ballylee mill. And how did she know that there was a mill here at all? Witchcraft wherever she got it; away she may have been in a trance" (1: 51). Another informant, the elderly Mr. Saggarton, even suggests that Early owned this cure and knew its exact location: "The cure for all things in the world? Surely she had it and knew where it was" (1: 97). Early searched in millstreams to collect some of the ingredients needed for cures. She also collected early-morning dew and, at times, instructed her patients to do the same. Daniel Shea, who went to Early in order to cure his supposedly fairy-stricken son, was told "to go out before sunrise to where there'd be a boundary wall between two or three estates, and to bring a bottle, and lay it in the grass and gather the dew into it" (1: 58). John Rainsford writes that moss was the substance that Early sought in millstreams[16]:

> [Early] used such ingredients as moss taken from a local mill stream, dandelions, seeds of flax, cat mint, turnips, thyme tea, nettles, potatoes, apples and honey for ailments like coughs, colds, wounds and scolds. Biddy gathered these ingredients before sun-up to ensure that the dew was still on them. This was reminiscent of earlier "Alchemists" who regarded dew as "a secretion from dawning light"—a key ingredient of the "Philosopher's Stone"—said to cure all ailments and to grant its owner eternal life. (45)

Yeats sought after the shade of Early as she gathered moss with the dew still on by the millstream of Ballylee at dawn. This image of the Celtic Twilight, from a woman and culture with its own distinctive cultural and medical practices, was what he attempted to capture.

* * *

[16] This information was found in John Rainsford's article, titled "Biddy Early's Limerick Connections" (2012), which is printed in the winter edition of *Old Limerick Journal* on pages 45–49. An electronic copy of this journal article can be found in the library archives on the Limerick City and County Council website: www.limerickcity.ie/Library/LocalStudies/BooksJournals/TheOldLimerickJournal/. Rainsford also published "Feakle's Biddy Early: a victim of 'moral panic'?" (2012) in *History Ireland*.

If, as Rainsford suggests, dawn-gathered moss had some of the properties of the philosophers' stone, then this chimes with Yeats's rooted desire, visible everywhere in his poetry, to avoid age, remain youthful, maintain health, and defy death. In Irish folklore, moss features in many beauty treatments and cures for ailments of the skin.[17] In the Battle of Clontarf, soldiers "stuffed their wounds with moss" due to its antiseptic nature (Ayres 28). It was revived as a treatment for injuries in the First World War (1914–1918), where it was recognised as an old Irish cure (Ayres 28). Historically, sphagnum moss preserved "bog bodies" due to its natural ability to prevent decay.[18] Yeats's poetry is replete with references to age and decrepitude; moss might preserve and renew an ageing and ailing human body.

Yeats sets "A Song of the Rosy Cross" (1891), a poem about "gain and loss" on the "wandering pathway" of life, in "a wood of dew and moss" (lines 1, 6, 5). Composed using trochaic heptamer, this one-stanza work was written on 15 November 1891, approximately six years prior to his arrival at Ballylee and his encounter with the old miller's story. The "dew and moss" combination speaks to Early's practice of collecting moss in rivers in Limerick, Clare, and Galway. Folk practices like these informed his thinking long before he came to Ballylee. By the time he arrived there, he was tuned to the idea that moss and dew could be salutary, even salvific, helping to preserve life, escape death, and thus avoid age.

Yeats's early knowledge of the place of moss in the cosmology of magical cures is evidenced in Lady Jane Wilde's "The Horned Women," first published in *Ancient Legends, Mystic Charms, and Superstitions of Ireland* (1887), her own collection of mainly spoken narratives and past beliefs.

[17] Moss is a herb of preservation and recovery; it carries qualities that help to sustain health and encourage the body to recover from illness. Patrick Logan states that "[t]here are, of course, a whole series of beauty treatments which form a part of Irish folk medicine" and that "[a] simple one is to rub the skin with the raw surface of a cucumber, which was done to remove freckles" (*Making the Cure* 76–77). On the subject of Irish moss, William Waldo Bauer claims in *Potions, Remedies, and Old Wives' Tales* (1969) that "[*c*]*ucumbers* found their way not only into the diet, where they belong, but to the cosmetic shelf in the form of skin lotions, often combined with Irish moss" (102). Logan further mentions that "bog moss is also used to treat a sprain" and "wounds were sometimes dressed with a moss found growing on human skulls which had been left exposed to the air" (*Making the Cure* 125, 89).

[18] Stuart McLean notes that Seamus Heaney wrote "The Grauballe Man" (1975), which is based on a bog body found in 1952 ("Bodies from the Bog" 299–300).

With only a few minor changes, Yeats reprinted Wilde's story in his early compendium of folklore, named *Fairy and Folk Tales of the Irish Peasantry* (1888).[19] A wealthy woman is instructed to "[t]ake yellow clay and moss, and bind them together, and plaster the sieve so that it will hold" (166). This moss contributes to the family being "restored" from some witches' enchantments (167).

Yeats was very likely to have later read about bygone cures, including moss and honey, in Lady Jane Wilde's *Ancient Cures, Charms, and Usages of Ireland* (1890). In total, moss is mentioned in Wilde's work five times; it is a cure for inflammation and blood loss (12; 40). It was thought that "[n]ine handfuls of mountain moss, dried on a pan to powder" forms part of a cure for inflammation; "the moss from a dead man's skull brought over from Ireland" was used to stop bleeding (Wilde 12, 40).[20] Wilde records a theory that robins built up moss around Jesus Christ in order to hide Him from His persecutors; the water-wagtail bird then removes this moss and thus betrays Him (61).[21] In "The Doctor's Visit," she writes about a medical doctor, who returns from the fairy world with a "handful of moss" that replaces the "golden guineas" (147). By the time Yeats first

[19] Lady Jane Wilde collected and wrote this folk tale; it features in Yeats's *Fairy and Folk Tales of the Irish Peasantry* (1888). In terms of minor changes: Yeats inserts two paragraph breaks, adds in three commas, employs one extra semi-colon, and removes the dash from "Slieve-namon" (Wilde, *Ancient Legends* 1: 18–21; Yeats, *Fairy and Folk Tales* 165–168). He also contributes a note to the piece, stating that "Slievenamon" is "*Sliábh-na-mban*—i.e., mountains of the women" (Yeats, *Fairy and Folk Tales* 167). Furthermore, he pluralises Wilde's singular use of "tree" and instead writes: "Open, open, wood and trees and beam!" (Wilde, *Ancient Legends* 1: 20; Yeats, *Fairy and Folk Tales* 167). He moves Wilde's sentence, "Take yellow clay and moss and bind them together and plaster the sieve so that it will hold," up to the above line and applies two commas so that it becomes, "Take yellow clay and moss, and bind them together, and plaster the sieve so that it will hold" (Wilde, *Ancient Legends* 1: 19; Yeats, *Fairy and Folk Tales* 166). He employs these commas in order to, both visually and grammatically, bind the ingredients together through punctuation. Yeats thought of moss as a material that could be used to weave ingredients together; likewise, moss and millstreams and Early are associated with each other.

[20] Wilde's cure for inflammation, containing the ingredient of moss, is set out as follows: "Nine handfuls of mountain moss, dried on a pan to powder. Nine pinches of it, and nine pinches of the ashes from the hearth, to be mixed in whey, taken every Tuesday and Thursday" (*Ancient Cures* 12).

[21] Wilde adds that, because of this act, the water-wagtail bird has "been considered unholy and unlucky, while the robin is held sacred, and no one would dare to injure it" (*Ancient Cures* 61).

heard the tale of Early's healing moss or herb from the miller in 1896, he was well primed by his reading to see the magical significance in such things.

* * *

The mossy millboards where Early gathered her healing materials are a key component of Thoor Ballylee. Yeats renovated this tower, according to a letter to John Quinn, using "contents of an old mill—great beams and three-inch planks, and old paving stones" (qtd. in Wade, *Letters* 651).[22] The three drafts of Yeats's "To be Carved on a Stone at Thoor Ballylee" (1921), which mention these boards, metamorphose from curse to blessing. Just as the tower's honeybees could either sting or store, witches can either curse or cure. In his successive redraftings, Yeats leaves witch-like premonitions on a healing instead of a cursing note, and literally sets the final draft in stone to secure its permanence. In total, there are three successive drafts of "To be Carved on a Stone at Thoor Ballylee," which are presented below[23]:

William Yeats & his wife George
With smithy work from the Gort forge
And wood from Coole & good brown sedge
Restored this Tower. They call a curse

[22] Yeats wrote about the building materials that he purchased for Thoor Ballylee in his correspondence with art collector John Quinn. Yeats wrote this letter on 23 July 1918, and he addressed it as "*Ballylee Castle* [/] *Gort, Co. Galway*" (qtd. in Wade, *Letters* 651).

[23] Joseph M. Hassett states that the early draft appears in Yeats's letter, dated on 23 July 1918, for John Quinn ("What Raftery Built" 97). He mentions another draft that was "preserved inside the plastic cover of a Cuala Press volume in the possession of Michael Yeats," and he references *Michael Robartes and the Dancer Manuscript Materials* as a source for this information (Hassett 103; Parkinson and Brannen 200). Hassett further notes that the last draft is found within the 1921 collection titled *Michael Robartes and the Dancer* (103). Hassett refers to an additional draft that he found in Parkinson and Brannen's *Michael Robartes and the Dancer: Manuscript Materials*, whereby "[b]oth Rafferty and the heirs appear in a handwritten text by a writer (other than Yeats) who counted the number of letters in each line, apparently with a view toward the carving of the lines on a stone" (Hassett 103; Parkinson and Brannen 198–99). The unknown writer rearranges parts of the poem, including the second line, which he changes to "With wood from Coole & broken slates" (qtd. in Parkinson and Brannen, 198–99). This version is not included in my study, as it was not penned in Yeats's hand but that of another writer. There are three known drafts of "To be Carved on a Stone at Thoor Ballylee" that Yeats definitely wrote himself.

On him who alters for the worst[24]
From fashion or a vulgar mind
What Rafferty built & Scott designed. (Undated; estimated circa. October–July 1918)[25]

* * *

I the poet William Yeats,
With common sedge and broken slates
And smithy work from the Gort forge
Restored this tower for my wife George;
And on my heirs I lay a curse
If they should alter for the worse,
From fashion or an empty mind,
What Rafftery built and Scott designed. (23 July 1918)

* * *

I, the poet William Yeats,
With old mill boards and sea-green slates,
And smithy work from the Gort forge,
Restored this tower for my wife George;
And may these characters remain
When all is ruin once again. (1921)

The curse only survives in the first two drafts; "They call a curse / On him who alters for the worst" moves to "And on my heirs I lay a curse / If they should alter for the worse" to then, as if by magic, disappear into thin air at the arrival of the third draft. The curse metamorphoses into a blessing

[24] Parkinson and Brannen note that the alternative word to "worst" is "worse" (200).

[25] Although undated, this version is likely to be Yeats's first draft; it was found in a Cuala Press book that his son (Michael Yeats) had inherited. This is because it acknowledges his wife's support with restoring Thoor Ballylee, which included financial contribution. Another reason to justify this version as Yeats's possible first draft is its style. In comparison to his two proceeding drafts, it is premature in the sense that his grand entrance as the poet is absent: "I, the poet William Yeats" (line 1). The letter containing the epitaph, written to the art and manuscript collector John Quinn on 23 July 1918, is therefore likely to have been the second draft. This leaves the publication in *Michael Robartes and the Dancer* (1921) as the third and final draft. Furthermore, Parkinson and Brannen list the poems in this order as well: they display unknown writer's version first, and then the three drafts that Yeats wrote with his own hand (198–200).

that hopes that "these characters remain / When all is ruin once again." Similarly, healing is a precursor to brokenness in so far as the "wood from Coole & good brown sedge" turn into "common sedge and broken slates" and finally are reimagined as "old mill boards and sea-green slates."[26]

Whilst writing the third draft, Yeats recalls the millboards, which carry a patina of associations with Early and the healing moss. Both physically and symbolically, Early is embodied in the building itself through the construction materials, the poetic voice, and the healing moss that weaves these ingredients together. Not only are the millboards part of the tower, their presence is signalled on a carved stone and in a printed book. These millboards have associations that bring Yeats back to his earliest days in Ballylee and, further, to the magical folk culture of the area. They have helped to restore his tower; the tower will restore a fractured world.

* * *

If the moss of the millboards might contain magical healing properties, so might the honey produced by the tower's bees. The famous bees of "The Stare's Nest by My Window" has long been a focus for many scholars. Whilst a significant number of critics have examined this poem, the honeybees' link to the healing properties of honey has gone unnoticed. In "The Honey-Bees of W. B. Yeats' 'The Stare's Nest at My Window': Echoes of Orpheus" (1979), Lee M. Whitehead proposed that the honeybee references in Yeats's "The Stare's Nest by My Window" are an

[26] In naming millboards, "sea-green slates" and "smithy work," Yeats joins the elements of wood, water, and fire, proposing that the tower is a place where the differing aspects of creation are unified (lines 2–3). The fire and water that Yeats associates with his wooden millboards feature heavily in Wilde's *Ancient Cures*. For example, when describing the beliefs of "[t]he Early Races," Wilde writes, "Fire was to them the sacred symbol of the divine essence, ever striving towards ascension; and water, ever seeking a level, was the emblem of the purification that should cover all daily life; while in the elemental earth they reverenced the power that produces all things, and where all that lives finds a grave, yet also a resurrection" (1). This applies to Yeats and his millboards because, whilst finding a place (Thoor Ballylee) for the fragments of Irish heritage to rest in peace, he is simultaneously resurrecting them back into the living world. However, even though Yeats's first draft of "To be Carved on a Stone at Thoor Ballylee" contains a curse, Yeats uses fire and water as curers in the third draft by including the millboards—which are an amalgamation of wood, fire, and water in themselves.

"allusion to the myth of Orpheus" (55).[27] Later on, in his Nobel Prize acceptance speech in 1995, the Irish poet Seamus Heaney discussed the contrast between the readers' "sympathetic nature" in "unsympathetic" environments ("Crediting poetry").[28] In the online article "Escaping Lockdown with W. B. Yeats" (2020), Joseph M. Hassett wrote that "[t]he honey-bees seem almost to have been willed into existence as an antidote to bitterness, unhappiness and uncertainty" and that "[r]eplacing bitter political fantasies with bee-like co-operation is the path to sweetness and light." It is interesting that Aristaeus's bees are produced through "begonia" (out of an animal carcass), thus foreshadowing Yeats's desire for honey to be generated in the unpropitious, murderous times in which his poem is composed.[29] Honey was viewed as medicinal in antiquity too. Therefore, much attention has been given to the honeybees in relation to the political climate, but their relationship to medicine has been overlooked.

Yeats owned an English prose edition of *Virgil*, as he spoke no Latin.[30] Those later bees of Yeats in "The Stare's Nest by My Window" would seem to recall the earlier bees in the distinctly pastoral poem "In the Seven Woods" (1903), where they are associated with Gregory's Coole Park. Yeats would have read about the "Hyblæan bees about your hedges taste / The flowering willows," how the "[b]alm-crickets feed on dew and bees on thyme," "the sound / Of birds" that "is in the amorous air, and bees," and the "[w]ild-thyme of bees" (Virgil 21, 56, 87–88, 94).[31] The story of Aristaeus's bees in the *Fourth Georgic* (c. 42–37 BCE)—which includes

[27] This is because the honeybee stories in Yeats's poetry and Virgil's *Fourth Georgic* look at "the necessity of descent into disorder and destruction, out of which 'all things are built again'" (Whitehead 55). This is a reference to Yeats's "Lapis Lazuli," in which poem he writes that "[a]ll things fall and are built again" (line 35). Whitehead writes, "But if we recall a story about bees, which also concerns Orpheus, in Virgil's Fourth Georgic, we might see that there is no contradiction in these implications of the image of the honey-bees; the story suggests that order, harmony, clarity, peace, emerge in the order of things by the metamorphosis of disorder, intoxication …" (57).

[28] Heaney postulates that Yeats "began to associate the sight of a mother feeding its young with the image of the honey bee, an image deeply lodged in poetic tradition and always suggestive of the ideal of an illustrious, harmonious, nurturing commonwealth" ("Crediting Poetry").

[29] In mythology, Aristaeus was a Greek god that founded beekeeping.

[30] In *A Descriptive Catalog of W. B. Yeats' Library* (1985), Edward O'Shea references Yeats's copy of *Virgil* as such: "Virgil. An English Version of the Eclogues of Virgil. Translated by Samuel Palmer. Illustrated by Samuel Palmer. London: Seeley, 1883" (293).

[31] These quotations are taken from *An English Version of the Eclogues of Virgil* (1883), which is the edition that Yeats himself owned and stored in his library.

the tale of Orpheus and Eurydice as an inset story—does indeed deploy the bees as an image of creativity and order. Virgil's is also (like Yeats's) a Civil War poem desiring order in seeming chaos. The beekeeping founder and mythological Greek god, Aristaeus, tends to the bees that become ill. Through altar-building and animal sacrifice, healthy bees arise from the carcasses of the deceased cattle:

> … He, as his mother bade,
> So does at once; without delay repairs
> To the Nymphs' shrines, the altars due prepares,
> Leads forth four bulls of noblest form and size,
> …
> Scarce ended this, when, strange to tell, they see,
> Amaz'd a sudden, wondrous, prodigy,
> Through the decaying vitals of each steer,
> From all its carcase and burst sides appear
> Bees buzzing, now like some vast clouds they form,
> Rock to and fro, now on some tree-top swarm; …
> These lays I sang about the care of bees,
> Of fields, of flocks and herds, of plants and trees, … (Virgil, *Fourth Georgic* 74–75)[32]

Bees are presented as being empathetic with humanity in their times of illness in so far as: "With sore disease / If they grow weak,—and life afflicts the bees / And us alike," and they are also associated with moss as "the hive" is "edg'd round / With moss" (Virgil 36, 2).[33] Brian Arkins and Warwick Gould have produced work on Yeats's use of *Virgil*. In *Builders of My Soul: Greek and Roman Themes in Yeats* (1990), Brian Arkins states that "Yeats's debt to Virgil is the opposite of that to Catullus: instead of a generalized influence, it is here the influence of one poem that is paramount, the *Fourth Eclogue*" (143). In the same vein, Warwick Gould, in "Lips and Ships, Peers and Tears: *Lacrimae Rerum* and Tragic Joy" (2013), postulates that Yeats's "war poetry, in particular, is nourished by a classical frame of reference, however modern, local and intimate the details

[32] This quotation is taken from the translator R. M. Millington's edition of Virgil's *Fourth Georgic*, titled *The Fourth Georgic of Virgil, Containing an Account of the Treatment of Bees, the Story of Aristaeus and His Bees, the Episode of Orpheus and Eurydice; and an Article on the Gladiator* (1870).

[33] These quotations are also taken from the translator R. M. Millington's edition of *The Fourth Georgic of Virgil* (1870).

of its horror" (16). Virgil's pastoral Civil War poem *Fourth Georgic*, which relays Greek beekeeping legend, was written in the bracket of 42–37 BCE (as with his other *Eclogues*). The war poem genre and the birth of sweet bees from chaos speaks to Yeats's treatment of the wounded world at the time, which he sought to medicate through his literary works that included his knowledge of folk remedies.

Whilst moss occupies much of Yeats's thinking, honey serves as a sweeter organic metaphor for healing, revival, and restoration. The therapeutic aspects of honey are extensive in traditional Irish medicine. Patrick Logan noted in his book, *Making the Cure: A Look at Irish Folk Medicine* (1972), that mixtures containing honey were used to treat common colds and chest problems (27).[34] Like moss, honey is also a natural substance that was used to help bind other ingredients together.[35] In a remedy designed to melt stones (such as gallstones and kidney stones), honey is included in order "to sweeten the mixture which is strained and bottled" (Logan 38).[36] The County Leitrim cure for aphthous ulcers "was to swab them with a mixture of honey and borax" (Logan 53). For eczema treatment, honey is "mixed with thick buttermilk" and applied to the affected skin (Logan 72). Logan notes that "mel saponis (honey of soap)" was a poultice, which he "think[s] has now been banished from the pharmacopoeia" at his time of writing, used to extract infection from boils (106). Honey also acted "as a dressing to protect boils and excoriations" (Logan 106). It is both a soother and a sweetener; at a difficult time, Yeats learns to metaphorically honey glaze his personal and health problems in order to make them easier to swallow.

Yeats would have gained some of his knowledge of honey, like moss, from his copy of Lady Wilde's *Ancient Cures*. These Irish lore contributions list honey as a cure for sore eyes, blindness, head pain, madness, falling sickness, and deafness (28–29, 33–34, 39, 42). In order to cure sore eyes, it was thought that the "yarrow, and honey, and the gall of fish boiled together and strained, then applied to the eye, will carry off every

[34] Logan notes that "[a]ll the usual mixtures, already mentioned, were used to treat colds; egg white; honey; linseed oil; sugar and mulled stout, etc." (27).

[35] For example, Logan states that "[o]ne rather elaborate mixture contained honey to which lemon juice had been added and all cooked into a thick paste with flour" (27).

[36] Logan is referring to a traditional County Galway remedy for gallstones, which was to ensure that "the roots of butchers' broom are boiled for eight hours and a pint of whiskey added to the quart of the water" (38). Logan writes that one of his informants says, "It melts the kidney stone and every stone in your body" (38).

description of blindness and clear the pains of the head" (Wilde 29). As they are "not procured by human means" and "not made by the hand of man," "honey, milk, and salt" were a cure for madness if this concoction was administered to the patient "to drink before sunrise in a sea-shell" (Wilde 34). In Wilde's discussion of the falling sickness, she paraphrases medical instructions from Thomas Joseph Pettigrew, a nineteenth-century surgeon (39–40). In his book, *On Superstitions Connected with the History and Practice of Medicine and Surgery* (1844), he wrote about the great powers that were attributed to herbs gathered after "an expiatory sacrifice of fruit and honey," which would give them the "power to render the possessor invulnerable, to cure fevers, to eradicate poison, and to conciliate friendship" (39). Yeats would have been aware of honey's therapeutic effects and its long history as an iatric substance.

In "The Stare's Nest by My Window," the sixth section of "Meditations in Time of Civil War" within *The Tower* collection (1928), the refrain is an imperative command directed at the honey-bees: "Come build in the empty house of the stare" (lines 5, 10, 15, 20). Whereas the first four lines of each stanza relay the brokenness that emanates from the Irish Civil War (1922–1923), the longer final line is consistent, reliable, and signifies recovery:

> The bees build in the crevices
> Of loosening masonry, and there
> The mother birds bring grubs and flies.
> My wall is loosening; honey-bees,
> Come build in the empty house of the stare.
>
> We are closed in, and the key is turned
> On our uncertainty; somewhere
> A man is killed, or a house burned,
> Yet no clear fact to be discerned:
> Come build in the empty house of the stare.
>
> A barricade of stone or of wood;
> Some fourteen days of civil war;
> Last night they trundled down the road
> That dead young soldier in his blood:
> Come build in the empty house of the stare.
>
> We had fed the heart on fantasies,
> The heart's grown brutal from the fare;
> More substance in our enmities

Than in our love; O honey-bees,
Come build in the empty house of the stare. (lines 1–20)

The birds and the honeybees are building back up the parts of the wall that have been lost and broken, which mirrors how Yeats hopes for a healing of the divisions in a fractured Ireland. The language of this poem is powerfully evocative of injury for Yeats as an individual and Ireland as a whole. The "dead young soldier in his blood," placed in the third stanza, is a poignant symbol of war casualties. In the final stanza, Yeats writes about having "fed the heart on fantasies" so that the "heart's grown brutal from the fare." The injury-heavy imagery of the poem reflects a time that left the Irish heart damaged; people were physically or emotionally injured, sometimes both. The Easter Rising (1916) was fresh in the minds of Irish people, and the world was still reeling from the effects of the First World War (1914–1918). Yeats acknowledges both bodily and spiritual trauma, but he also applies a moss and honey-like effect to the world's wounds.

Yeats's "The Stare's Nest by My Window" reprises deeply laid ideas in relation to honey in his work. In "The Lake of Innisfree" (1893), one of his earliest celebrated poems, Yeats longs to "have some peace" and embark on a less grand building project than his tower in the form of "a small cabin build there, of clay and wattles made" (lines 5, 2). Beside this house he wishes to have "a hive for the honey-bee" and to "live alone in the bee-loud glade" and hear the lake water "in the deep heart's core" (lines 3, 4, 12). In *The Celtic Twilight*, he describes "unreason" as "ready for the wild bees of truth to hive in it, and make their sweet honey" (*Mythologies* 442). In this passage, the similarity to the wording of "The Stare's Nest by My Window" is striking: "Come into the world again, wild bees, wild bees!" (442).

In Yeats's *The Countess Cathleen*, a famine play whereby the eponymous protagonist rescues the local Irish people, Cathleen stops and poses the question: "Surely this leafy corner, where one smells / The wild bee's honey, has a story too?" (lines 291–92). Although the play was first published in 1892 and 1895, he added these lines about honey in 1899, when it was republished again as part of the third edition of his *Poems* (1899).[37] This was after his initial visits to Coole that began in August 1896, and which became an unfaltering tradition thereafter.

[37] Yeats continued to reprint *The Countess Cathleen*, maintaining his addition about the honeybees.

Much later, in an endnote to his Nobel Prize acceptance speech, *The Irish Dramatic Movement: A Lecture Delivered to the Royal Academy of Sweden* (1924), Yeats writes that, amid the bloodshed of the Irish Civil War, "[o]ne felt an overmastering desire not to grow unhappy or embittered, not to lose all sense of the beauty of nature" (*Autobiographies* 523).[38] Inspired by a stare that "had built in a hole beside my window," "The Stare's Nest by my Window" was constructed "out of the feeling of the moment" (523). During this process, Yeats reports an epiphanic experience: "Presently a strange thing happened. I began to smell honey in places where honey could not be, at the end of a stone passage or at some windy turn of the road, and it came always with certain thoughts" (523).[39] In other words, Yeats is finding positivity in the darkest of situations, symbolised by the "stone passage" end and the "windy turn of the road" that simulates life's unpredictable and transient nature. References to honey are stored throughout his poems, plays, folk tales, and autobiographies.[40] The smell of honey came with thoughts that he could not be consumed by hatred; honey is associated with recovery from acrimony. Directly following his enlightening moment, Yeats refers to his experience in Dublin, where he "was with angry people who argued over everything or were eager to know the exact facts" (523). This passage encapsulates Yeats's

[38] Yeats delivered his Nobel Prize speech, *The Irish Dramatic Movement: A Lecture Delivered to the Royal Academy of Sweden*, on 15 December 1923 and then published it in 1924.

[39] This quotation can be found in an endnote within *The Irish Dramatic Movement: A Lecture Delivered to the Royal Academy of Sweden* (*Autobiographies* 523). In this endnote, Yeats quotes his own poem that contains instances of honey. For example: "My wall is loosening; honey-bees" is a line from "The Stare's Nest by My Window" (523). The "windy turn of the road," that he uses to describe his epiphanic experience, could also symbolise Yeats's changing emotions in response to heartbreak and loss (523).

[40] In Yeats's *Autobiographies*, there are eight references to honey in total. The examples, that are not mentioned in the main part of this study, are as follows. In *Reveries Over Childhood and Youth* (1916), Yeats writes about a "too-honeyed verse" (*Autobiographies* 93). Another reference appears in "Book I: Four Years: 1887–1891" (1921) of *The Trembling of the Veil* (1922): "I had lived upon bread and tea because I thought that if antiquity found locust and wild honey nutritive, my soul was strong enough to need no better" (140). "Book II: Ireland After Parnell" (1922) inhabits two references to honey: "nearest the honeyed comb" and "he might have brought the imagination of Ireland nearer … the honeycomb" (174, 183). For his prepositional in "Book II: Ireland After Parnell" (1922), "nearest the honeyed comb," Yeats alludes to Judges 14.5–8 in the Bible in his paraphrase: "The biblical parable of bees and honey in the carcase; sweetness and light coming from terror and destruction" (*Autobiographies* 174, 459; *Holy Bible*).

revelation that to labour on the basis of resentment, bitterness, and indignation is futile. In being able to smell the honey, Yeats is open to inhaling a new life perspective. It is as if his senses have been revived and reinvigorated; he has experienced a realisation.

Honey is therefore a medical and metaphysical reliever of both bodily and emotional pain; Yeats is a practitioner of self-medication in so far as he adds the healing properties of honey to both his poetry and personal life. In "Seers and Healers," Gregory recalls a time when she brought Yeats to a healer around the Connemara area, Fagan, who confirmed that his "*uncertain eyesight*" was not the result of a fairy curse (103). Although Gregory does not mention that any prescription was given, honey was often employed to recover sight as well as fight other ailments (Wilde, *Ancient Cures* 29). In his poetry, Yeats used the idea of honey to restore his mind's sight and sweeten his thoughts with a more positive perception. This did not eradicate his problems, but changed his reaction to them, just as honey sweetens bitter-tasting medicine. In comparison to his long-term emotional reaction to heartbreak, Yeats adopted a collected attitude to the anger that surrounded him on his visit to Dublin in 1922.[41] Honey provided Yeats with a renewed sense of optimism.

As bees collect nectar in order to build and store honey, Yeats collects building materials and folklore with the view to storing them away in both his tower and his literary works. In "The Stare's Nest by My Window," Yeats writes about "[a] barricade of stone or of wood" in relation to the Civil War (line 11). The materials that constitute this barrier bring to mind the fabric of Thoor Ballylee, restored with stonework from the local mill and Coole wood, a sanctuary for the Yeats family, birds, and bees. In creating this correspondence between the materials of a hastily thrown-up barricade and his own venerable home, Yeats imbues his poem with the unspoken suggestion that the violence and bitterness of the present might one day be sweetened to a calm place where the honeybee might find shelter.

Honey was viewed in Irish folk medicine as a powerful curative, and Yeats applied this to his own life and work, the Irish language and folklore, as well as national and international wounds. In "The Sorcerers," a chapter in *The Celtic Twilight* (1902), Yeats investigates dark powers in the world as well as "bright beings who store their honey in the cells of [the

[41] This visit to Dublin in 1922 is detailed in an endnote within *The Irish Dramatic Movement: A Lecture Delivered to the Royal Academy of Sweden* (*Autobiographies* 523).

human] heart" (*Mythologies* 447). He similarly stores folklore in Thoor Ballylee, the core of his revival project, permitting the proceeding literary colony to continue Irish traditions. Bees pass on the honey to each other, and this emulates the folklore-gathering process: narratives are passed on and eventually stored more permanently through the written word.

After a long recovery from heartbreak and loss, it is the therapeutic aspects of honey that become his muse. Honey has a therapeutic effect on him in so far as its healing symbolism cures him from looking at situations with a bleak perspective. Although anger, arguments, and the hope for certainty are "in the midst of the mood that makes realistic drama," Yeats exposes these tensions as counterproductive to strong health (*Autobiographies* 523; "Notes"). Honey provides him with a new lens with which to view the world, the international space, the European landscape, Ireland, his relationships, and himself.

* * *

Yeats's tower is a place of healing and renewal on a personal and national level. Just as ligaments join bone to bone, Early is the connective tissue that links the folkloric, the occult, and medicine. Through their contact with her healing moss, the millboards with which Yeats restored the tower carry with them magical and salutary associations. Wilde's collection of cures, as read by Yeats himself, underscores moss as a therapeutic and magical substance in Irish folklore. Thoor Ballylee is not the only thing those millboards "cured"; just as Yeats patches up the tower, he simultaneously patches together the world's wounds. A practitioner in words rather than medicine, Yeats rebuilds Thoor Ballylee as an amalgamation of fractures that might, in being re-set, heal stronger. He fixes together national and international conflict as well as remedy the wider tensions at the heart of the Irish Revival: between Irish and English, the ancient and the new, the mystical and the scientific.

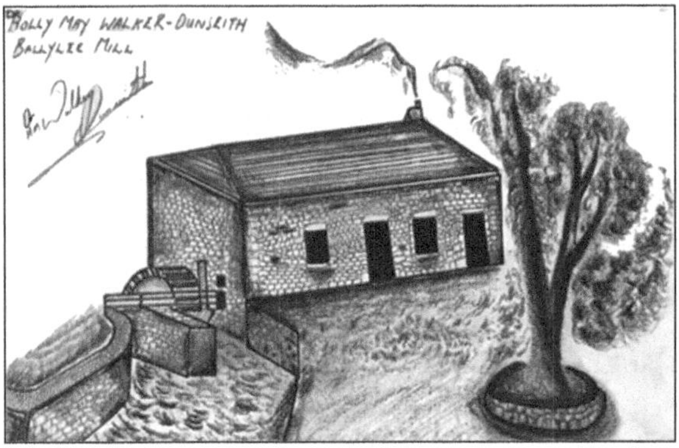

Ballylee Mill

PART II

Augusta Gregory: From Colonies to Cough Medicines

CHAPTER 4

Rejuvenation, Medicine, and Revival in the Works of Augusta Gregory

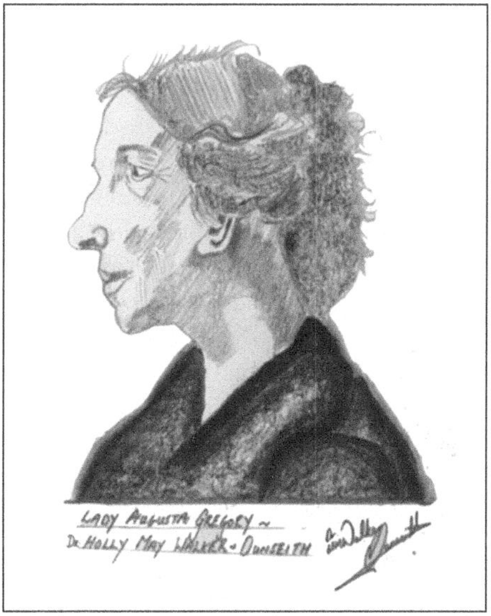

Lady Augusta Gregory

H. M. Walker-Dunseith, *Traditional Medicine in the Irish Literary Revival*, New Directions in Irish and Irish American Literature, https://doi.org/10.1007/978-3-031-82459-3_4

In the decade that followed the death of her husband, Sir William Gregory, in 1892, Augusta Gregory reinvented herself. In her act of self-redefinition, she selected new role models and guises for her life. With her collaborator W. B. Yeats she dramatised a spiritual self-portrait in the form of Cathleen Ni Houlihan, who walks away from the action, young again, at the end of the play of that name. This process of rejuvenation and self-reinvention was familiar to her collaborator, Yeats, who theorised that the poet is "reborn as an idea, something intended, complete" and who famously stated, "*It is myself that I remake*" (*Essays and Introductions* 509; "Untitled Poem" line 4). Gregory imagined her role as a dramatist and editor in medical terms: "I am rather a good play doctor," she wrote in a letter to writer Thomas Joseph Kiernan on 28 November 1928, when she was telling him that "I have been helping some of our authors—old & new—to get their plays right" (qtd. in New York Public Library, *Bulletin* 26). She imitated models and guides that she took from her locality: one was the folk healer Biddy Early. Another was Cathleen Ni Houlihan herself, the protagonist from the eponymous single-act play about a *cailleach* (the Irish word for a hag but also a sovereignty goddess associated with the territory of Ireland) who transforms from old to young.[1] This reinvented self and the state of being reborn is relevant at a national and personal level for Gregory. Biddy Early and Cathleen Ni Houlihan are linked together. According to Gearóid Ó Crualaoich, the *cailleach* is connected to the *bean feasa* or wise woman as well as "the *bean ghlúine* (midwife)" and "the *bean chaointe* (keening-woman)" (29). Both Biddy Early and Cathleen Ni Houlihan are forms of healer and when Gregory reinvented herself, the model of healing woman was one on which she drew.

In an outdoor production of *Cathleen Ni Houlihan* in 2020, staged at Coole Park itself, the Druid Theatre director Garry Hynes deliberately chose an actress to look like Gregory.[2] In an interview for the *Irish Women's Writing (1880–1920) Network* titled *In Conversation with Garry Hynes* (2021), she discusses her decision to cast actress Marie Mullen as a Gregory-lookalike Cathleen and expands upon the subtleties of Gregory's

[1] For information about the *cailleach*, see Robert Welch's *The Cold of May Day Monday: An Introduction to Irish Literature* (2014) and Gearóid Ó Crualaoich's *The Book of the Cailleach: Stories of the Wise Woman Healer* (2003).

[2] For information about this production, staged in 2020, browse the website: www.druid.ie (*Druid Theatre*).

role in the play.[3] Hynes states, "[I]n *Cathleen Ni Houlihan*, Marie played the main role and was deliberately designed to look like Lady Gregory and that was an act of homage to her rather than any kind of impersonation or whatever" (00:28:56–00:29:14; my transcription).[4] Hynes talks about the significance of "Coole itself" in relation to Gregory and the experience of "seeing the play but then ... journeying from that space to another space in Coole" which "just felt very connected to her" and she says that "there was a very real, very emotional connection with her" (00:28:30–52; 00:29:16–20; my transcription).[5] Although this casting choice is made to signify a public respect for Gregory and her work, there is a beacon of truth in the similarity between Cathleen Ni Houlihan and Gregory that stretches far beyond physical appearance.

The focus on healing in the literary career that began around her fortieth year had roots in her previous life. Gregory, in a letter she wrote to the anti-imperialist poet Wilfrid Scawen Blunt in March 1885, hinted that she had medicinal duties in her district. In her autobiography, *Seventy Years* (1974), she reproduces a letter in which this is apparent:

> We arrived here [i.e. Coole] two days ago, the weather is cold and even the horse-chestnut trees hardly give promise of a leaf (just three weeks behind Paris) and I was so tired by travelling and unpacking that I have not yet recovered my energy, but half dormant take up my old occupations and buy flannel and make cough cures for old women. But little Robert is bright enough for two and as happy as the day is long ... (Gregory 209; ellipsis in source)

[3] This interview was part of the *Collaborations and Networks Symposium 2021*, which "explored the various ways in which Irish women writers engaged in and developed diverse creative collaborations in order to produce a wide range of works" ("Collaborations and Networks Symposium 2021").

[4] This is a response to interviewer Anna Pilz's question: "What do you make of Coole Park as a site that has its own kind of social, historical, and political contexts and when you have then plays—both *Cathleen Ni Houlihan* [1902] and *The Rising of the Moon* [1907]; and *The Gaol Gate* [1900] actually—with very kind of nationalist overtones in that space . . . what does that do to the meaning of the plays?" (00:26:36–54; my transcription).

[5] Hynes states that "as a result of that, a play that Druid had been wanting to do for years, which is Tom Kilroy's version of *The Seagull* [1981], which he transplants to Celtic Revival Ireland in the 1890s" was performed in 2021 "in Coole Park on a stage and that, I must say, was haunted as well" (00:29:21–49; my transcription). She says, "to have a play which is about that period, to have the character of Kilroy's Constantine talk about plays that have roots that have meaning that have come from the voice of the people, to do that in Coole was, you know, the echoes were all over" (00:29:50-00:30:09; my transcription).

Over three years later, on 29 August 1888, Gregory wrote another letter to Blunt from Coole Park. In a similar style, this letter expanded upon her altruistic practices and, for all its wryness, ended on a positive note: "The poor people come to the door daily, believing that I can cure them of all diseases, including poverty, and I mix their cough-cures and buy their flannel and dye it with madder in an iron pot, and altogether I am at present one of the happy people without a history" (Gregory, *Seventy Years* 232).[6] Her claim to be "without a history" is an interesting one, as it is similar to the axiom—"Happy the people whose annals are blank in history books!"—which the Scottish historian Thomas Carlyle attributes to French philosopher Montesquieu.[7] This "history" whose existence is antithetical to happiness is worth dwelling on.

The fraught colonial and religious history of Gregory and Coole Park are ingredients that contribute to her past. Gregory was a Persse by birth; the descendent of a seventeenth-century Protestant preacher.[8] This ancestor of hers, Reverend Robert Persse, "arrived [in Ireland] from England, probably before 1602" (Kearney 2). His grandson, Reverend Dudley Persse, thrived amid the religious vicissitudes of his time and "held five profitable church appointments and received large land grants from Charles II and James II" (Kohfeldt 9). He built the family seat of Roxborough and so, notes Gregory's biographer Mary Lou Kohfeldt, "[t]he family fortune was thus founded on royal favor and tithes of Catholic tenants to a church they abhorred" (Kohfeldt 9). Gregory's sisters and mother may have proselytised in the Famine, which involved

[6] The idea that Gregory had the ability to cure people "of all diseases," however, ironically expressed, links Coole Park to the recovery of health, and to the elixir, something I discuss further in my chapter on W. B. Yeats ("Thoor Ballylee: Healing and Recovery"). The idea that this place might be one of all-healing is a recurrent one.

[7] Translator Marian Schwartz and editor Gary Saul Morson published an edition of Leo Tolstoy's *Anna Karenina* in 2014, which includes a footnote that explains the origins of this proverb: "In *War and Peace*, in a draft of *Anna Karenina*, and elsewhere, Tolstoy cites a French proverb: 'Happy people have no history.' [The Scottish historian Thomas] Carlyle attributes to [the French philosopher Charles-Louis de Secondat, baron de La Brède et de] Montesquieu: 'Happy the people whose annals are blank in history books!' The idea is that happy families resemble each other because they have no dramatic events worthy of a history, but unhappy families each have their own story" (743).

[8] In *Lady Gregory: The Woman Behind the Irish Renaissance* (1985), Mary Lou Kohfeldt states, "The great estate upon which she [Gregory] was born had been bought by her great-great-great-great-grandfather Dudley Persse, a successful and favored Church of Ireland clergyman, in the late seventeenth century" (9).

going from house-to-house and trying to convert people from Catholicism to Protestantism.[9] In 1880, she married Sir William Henry Gregory, who was the Governor of Ceylon for the East India Company. This English company, incorporated by royal charter on 31 December 1600, was "formed for the exploitation of trade with East and Southeast Asia and India" ("East India Company"; *Encyclopædia Britannica*). Given the anti-colonial bent of Scawen Blunt's ideas perhaps, for Gregory, to be "without a history" would have been happiness indeed.

To be without a history enables one to begin again, and this was what Gregory was in the process of doing. Her decade of transformation spanned from 1892 to 1902 and began with the death of her husband on 6 March 1892. A trip to Inisheer not long after his death provided a glimpse of the kind of new life that Gregory envisaged for herself. Gregory claimed that she "was quite happy" when she took shelter in a cottage in October 1893 at Inisheer, one of the Aran Islands in Galway Bay, where the residents spoke Irish and ate potatoes as their staple diet (qtd. in Kohfeldt 94).[10] This cottage was the binary opposite to Coole Park and, for Gregory, this change of location both reflected and nurtured a gradual change of mind. She perused Irish narratives and folk stories, sparked a friendship with Yeats in August 1896, and went from door to door collecting folklore at Coole Park.[11] Yeats, Edward Martyn, and Gregory discussed plans for a "Celtic Theatre" in late June 1897.[12] In summer 1897, a progressive plan was born to establish the Abbey Theatre in Dublin, which would open its doors on 27 December 1902. Her self-reinvention as a contributor to the indigenous culture of Ireland was nearing its completion at New Year in 1898 when, in a letter to Blunt, Gregory

[9] The Irish novelist George Moore propounds that Gregory was "an ardent soul gatherer in the days gone by but abandoned missionary work when she married" (qtd. in Tóibín 13).

[10] Kohfeldt states, "[I]n October 1893, before anyone else in the Irish Renaissance—[Gregory] went to the Aran Isles, the three islands twenty miles off the coast of Galway ... She was stormbound there for five days, living on potatoes in a cottage with people who hardly spoke English" (94).

[11] Gregory's reading material included George Borrow's *Lavengro* (1851), Douglas Hyde's *Beside the Fire* (1890), Jane Barlow's *Irish Idyls* (1892), and Emily Lawless's *Grania* (1892) (Kohfeldt 94; Tóibín 24).

[12] The Irish Literary Theatre's first production—Yeats's *The Countess Cathleen*—was on 8 May 1899, at The Ancient Concert Rooms, Dublin; the Abbey Theatre (the successor to the Irish Literary Theatre and the Irish National Theatre Society, the latter of which was founded on 1 February 1903) opened its doors on 27 December 1904, at what was formerly the Mechanics Institute.

confirmed, "My own life is happy now, and I *almost* say to the passing moment stay" (qtd. in Kohfeldt 122). Anna Pilz provides evidence to indicate that, at this point in Gregory's life, she showed "active support of the Catholic Church and the Catholic community" ("*'The Return to the People'*" 120).[13] Furthermore, in 1900, Gregory accepted a project that Yeats had turned down due to time constraints.[14] *Cuchulain of Muirthemne: the Story of the Men of the Red Branch of Ulster*, a narrative and composite work based on the stories of the Ulster Cycle and other materials, was printed as a result in April 1902. Despite her grandeur and class, Gregory was, with Yeats, behind the incendiary nationalist play *Cathleen Ni Houlihan*, first performed in the same year. This controversial play did much to break down her old inherited image as an Anglo-Irish landowner.

This image of the occupant of a Big House dispensing medicine to the occupants of surrounding cottages, which appears in her letters of 1885 and 1888, is in some ways paradigmatic of colonialism, an image of a benign Big House landowner ministering to her dependent tenantry. Coole House, often referred to as the Big House, was an edifice built on the profits of exploitation. Gregory's grandfather-in-law, Robert Gregory, was an East India Company director. He purchased Coole Park from the Martyns in 1768, a wealthy family that owned much land in the area, using lucre from his work in India. This money also funded the construction of the house there in approximately 1770, which was therefore built on the foundations of colonialism. This was the same year as the Bengal Famine of 1770. Cormac Ó Gráda identifies this "poorly documented famine" as one of the "colonial famines" that was "the product of the East India Company's rapacity" ("Revisiting the Bengal Famine of 1943–4" 36). Nani Gopal Chaudhuri reports "the effects of the famine on population, land and silk and cotton industries" (239). William Dalrymple highlights that "the rural artisans and the urban poor, unprotected and with no safety net, were the first to sicken from malnutrition, then, one by one, to begin dying from starvation or disease" (216). This further exacerbated as "[b]y February 1770, when around 70 per cent of the usual rice crop had been lost, and the price of rice was ten times its normal rate, the hunger

[13] Amongst other examples that are detailed in Pilz's study, Gregory "worked hand in hand" with "the Sisters of Mercy" and "also with Catholic representatives of the upper class" ("*'The Return to the People'*" 120).

[14] Kohfeldt states, "In the summer of 1900 Yeats told her [Gregory] an English publisher had suggested he retell the Irish epics but he had refused because he didn't have the time" (139).

started to become much more widespread" (Dalrymple 216). This was the "history" that she was happy when she imagined herself without. As for James Joyce's Stephen Dedalus, the protagonist in *Ulysses* (1922), "[h]istory" was "a nightmare from which" Gregory was "trying to awake" (34).

Gregory's desired state of forgetfulness echoes the experiences of other colonists. The wife of Wilfrid Scawen Blunt, Lady Anne Blunt, wrote a travel work, *Pilgrimage to Nejd* (1881), about venturing to Arabia that was edited by her husband. Sinéad Garrigan Mattar identifies a passage in this *Pilgrimage to Nejd* that corresponds with the letter that Gregory wrote "[a] decade later" in which she denied her history ("'Wage for Each People Her Hand Has Destroyed'" 54). Mattar quotes a passage by Anne Blunt in this article, though I have restored passages that Mattar omits from the original source:

> DAMASCUS, Dec. 6, 1878.—It is strange how gloomy thoughts vanish as one sets foot in Asia. Only yesterday [5 December 1878] we were still tossing on the sea of European thought, with its political anxieties, its social miseries and its restless aspirations ... and now we seem to have ridden into still water, where we can rest and forget and be thankful. The charm of the East is the absence of intellectual life there, the freedom one's mind gets from anxiety in looking forward or pain in looking back. Nobody here thinks of the past or the future, only of the present; and till the day of one's death comes, I suppose the present will always be endurable. (qtd. in Mattar 54; Mattar's addition; ellipsis in the aforementioned source; *Pilgrimage to Nejd* 1: 1–2)

As Mattar observes, "when Gregory would describe to Blunt her own escape from a sea of troubles (primarily her ongoing love for him) in the primitive, non-intellectual present tense of the peasantry, she shifted the scene of this idyll easily from East to West" (54–55). The affair with the anti-colonial Wilfrid Scawen Blunt, which lasted a year and ended in 1883, is a sinister part of Gregory's "conversion" and happened much earlier than her decade of transformation that traversed from 1892 to 1902.

Anne Blunt's and Gregory's eternal presents are intriguing instances of an aspect of Edward W. Said's definition of Orientalism. This is a concept that Said coined in his book titled *Orientalism* (1978) which is, in editor Vincent B. Leitch's words, "focused particularly on imperialism and the interplay between the dominant West (the 'Occident') and the Middle and

Far East (the 'Orient')" (*Norton Anthology* 1986). Leitch further states, "For Said, the 'margin' of the East helps define the colonial center of the West, and the Oriental 'Other' is a projection of the Western view that constructs it" (1988). Said defines Orientalism as having a three-tiered meaning: it is "a way of coming to terms with the Orient that is based on the Orient's special place in European Western experience," it is "a style of thought based upon an ontological and epistemological distinction made between 'the Orient' and (most of the time) 'the Occident,'" and it is "a Western style for dominating, restructuring, and having authority over the Orient" (*Norton Anthology* 1991, 1992).[15] Said argues that "the Orient is an idea that has a history and a tradition of thought, imagery, and vocabulary that have given it reality and presence in and for the West" and "[t]he two geographical entities thus support and to an extent reflect each other" (1994). Gregory seemingly desired a present-tense perspective for her personal history in Ireland.

As the 1890s wear on, the nature of Gregory's self-reinvention becomes more apparent from her diaries and letters. When she wrote letters to Blunt, describing her healing panacea and happiness and history, she was addressing a catalyst who she later became. In April 1897, she created a diary entry that had a similar style to these letters. After returning to Coole from London, Gregory journaled, "Even with R. [her son, Robert Gregory] I feel a little chill coming back to the grey silence & the small cares — But that will pass away in service for others — & I feel much for the people, not able to sow their crops —" (*Lady Gregory's Diaries* 146). There is evidence here of an ethos that saw happiness in the self-forgetfulness that came from labour for less privileged people. By 1897, there is the hint that what was once a regular duty has become an inspiring vocation.

Long before Yeats became her neighbour in 1917, when he purchased Thoor Ballylee after negotiating its purchase throughout 1916, he exhibited medical complaints that rendered him dependent on Gregory's care. In a letter to Yeats, perhaps written in 1901, Gregory gives her patient some medical advice for his rheumatism: "How bad of you to get ill just

[15] He states, "[T]he Orient has helped to define Europe (or the West) as its contrasting image, idea, personality, experience" and "[y]et none of this Orient is merely imaginative" because "[t]he Orient is an integral part of European *material* civilization and culture" (*Norton Anthology* 1991). Said argues that "Orientalism expresses and represents that part culturally and even ideologically as a mode of discourse with supporting institutions, vocabulary, scholarship, imagery, doctrines, even colonial bureaucracies and colonial styles" (1991).

when I am not there to look after you! Do take care of yourself now, and feed yourself properly – and with any threatening of rheumatism you should look to your underwear" (qtd. in Tóibín 83–84). Prior to 1850, doctors recommended that underclothing should be made of flannel (Nunn 138). Maire Horgan, a collector for *The Schools' Manuscript Collection* (*NFCS*) in County Kilkenny, recorded that "[p]eople who suffered from rheumatic pains, often wore a red flannel undershirt, because red flannel is supposed to hold a cure for rheumatism" ("Local Cures" 512).[16] In Irish folklore, red flannel holds an inherent cure that works when the patient wears it beside their skin; no other colour would suffice. Folklore collector Helen Cooney, who lives in County Westmeath, writes: "[i]nside garments made of red flannel were worn as a remedy for rheumatism" ("Local Cures" 111).[17] Patrick Logan explains that the red flannel was also applied to whooping cough and sprains because "red is the colour used to expel demons" (*Making the Cure* 44, 124). Maureen Hurley, a collector in County Westmeath, attests to its "curative properties" and advises that "[p]eople who have a tendency to rheumatics should thatch their bodies with red flannel" ("Cures" 406).[18] This traditional Irish belief would explain the madder dye that Gregory writes about using on flannel. Gregory mirrors Yeats, and vice versa, as friends with similar medical interests that reflect the healing properties of the locality. Gregory perhaps reminding Yeats to wear flannel underclothing that has been dyed with red madder is a command that aims to restore both Yeats and the old folk medical practices of Ireland that she was continually learning about from the people around her.

Gregory dedicated the Irish edition of *Cuchulain of Muirthemne* (1902) to people living in the nearby Kiltartan parish. Her introduction is testament to her self-reinvention, though is marked by a distinct tonal oddity: "And indeed if there was more respect for Irish things among the learned men that live in the college at Dublin, where so many of these old writings are stored, this work would not have been left to a woman of the house, that has to be minding the place, and listening to complaints, and dividing her share of food" (vi). This is a slightly uncomfortable act of ventriloquism as Colm Tóibín perceives that "[t]he page-long

[16] *NFCS* 0865: 512; Collector: Maire Horgan (12), Clinstown (school), County Kilkenny, c. 1937-1939. Teacher: S. Ó Dúnlaing.

[17] *NFCS* 0722: 111; Collector: Helen Cooney, Carpenterstown (Templefanum) (school), Carpenterstown, County Westmeath, c. 1937–1939. Teacher: Mary Smyth.

[18] *NFCS* 0732: 406; Collector: Maureen Hurley, Kilbeggan (Mercy Convent) (school), Kilbeggan, County Westmeath, January 1938–January 1939. Teacher: Sr Philomena.

introduction managed a number of astonishing false notes, as though Lady Gregory had been caught halfway in the act of self-invention" (41). There is something uncanny about her writing in the voice of a peasant. She was not speaking from the mouth of a character but she was writing using her own voice to address the people who lived in Kiltartan, a civil parish and barony in County Galway. She ended the dedication by saying that they "have been very kind to me ever since I came over to you from Kilchriest, two-and-twenty years ago" (Gregory, *Cuchulain of Muirthemne* vi). Tóibín deduces that "[f]or a moment, Roxborough, with its English colonial sound, was being wiped off the map" and "[t]he place she came from, in this final sentence, would have an Irish name" (41). In this act of being reborn, Gregory is coming from a new place.

Why do we not, however, consider Gregory as a modernist? There is a more sympathetic way in Gregory's writing that might be, in Ezra Pound's words, "mak[ing] it new."[19] She is writing in an unexpected and superior way, but this may be a dangerous assumption. Gregory's Kiltartanese—like Synge's Hiberno-English—is "modernist" in its synthetic "primitivism." The French poet Tristram Corbière was using Breton to similar ends in the nineteenth century, where he was heavily drawing on the language. These are all instances of drawing on the Celtic fringes and margins to European and imperial modernity.

Yeats is prevalent in modernist scholarship; Gregory is absent. In his chapter titled "Austin Clarke: The Poet as Scapegoat of Modernism," W. J. McCormack argues that "[a]lthough the Irish contribution to Anglophone modernism was disproportionately large, efforts to define (or even comprehensively describe) the modernist movement have rarely engaged with the issue of national, regional or local provenance" and "[s]imilarly, schemes by which modernism in general has been periodized into early and late phases have paid little attention to the manner in which paleo-modernism depends heavily upon the pioneering work of Yeats in the 1890s *and* ignored the extent to which a 'neo-modernism' in the 1930s requires the existence of Beckett" (75).[20] After composing a list of Irish writers born between 1900 and 1907, McCormack argues that "only

[19] The phrase "[m]ake it new" was popularised as a modernist term by American poet Ezra Pound in his book *Make It New: Essays* (1934).

[20] McCormack writes, "Even if the detection of literary generations is fraught with imprecision, it is fair to say that in Samuel Beckett (*b.* 1906), John Hewitt (*b.* 1907), Denis Johnston (*b.* 1901), Louis MacNiece (*b.* 1907), Seán O'Faoláin (*b.* 1900), a new phase of literary endeavour was seen to follow on from that which had powerfully collected round Yeats (*b.* 1865), Synge (*b.* 1871), and Joyce (*b.* 1882)" ("Austin Clarke" 76–77).

Beckett and Johnston could be plausibly linked with the modernist movement" and "[n]ot only a preference for experimentation in literary form, but a willingness to confront the agreed order of things generally, differentiates them from writers (as different from each other as Hewitt and O'Faoláin) who still nurtured hopes of reconciliation with their societies and / or an improvement in those societies as such" (77). Gregory's modernism began with Kiltartanese at a local level and expanded as her work grew in other parts of Ireland; she both challenged and subverted issues that affected Ireland (such as colonialism) to remedy and heal societal wounds.

In his chapter "Against Irish Studies: Reading Austin Clarke and His Critics," on the other hand, John McAuliffe "concentrate[s] on the misleading critical reception of his 1929 volume of poetry, *Pilgrimage*, which reception has imposed a limit on the way in which his poetry is read, anthologized and taught, that is, the misleading critical representation of Clarke as a Gaelic poet, writing in the shadow of W. B. Yeats" (255). This same Irish poet, Austin Clarke, in a letter to poet Seumas O'Sullivan that was written on 23 August, possibly in 1935, "refers to the Irish Literary Revival as a baby abandoned by Yeats, which he and [American editor and writer] Joseph Campbell, finding the foundling on their doorstep, felt obliged to look after" (McAuliffe 257; Harmon 76, 262). McAuliffe infers that "[t]his obviously ties in with Yeats' idea of himself as primogenitor and first father of the Irish literary tradition" (257). If Yeats considered himself to be the Irish literary tradition's earliest father, then Gregory is the mother who also nurtures the Revival and teaches this "baby" to speak to the nation in Irish and Kilartanese.

Gregory's family played a role in proselytism as they had a controversial history of trying to convert people to Protestantism. George Moore, an Irish novelist who was not always the most reliable of witnesses, accused her of being "an ardent soul gatherer in the days gone by" who then "abandoned missionary work when she married" (qtd. in Tóibín 13). This refers to her teenage years in Roxborough, when members of the Persse family engaged in converting the local people. In response, Gregory admitted that "[m]y mother and my two eldest sisters ... made no secret of this proselytism which was much mixed up with benevolence and charity in those days" and that "my sister, Mrs. Shawe-Taylor, especially, worked ardently for its accomplishment" (qtd. in Tóibín 13–14). However, Gregory strongly denied her own participation in this conversion practice as she claims that "I myself, the youngest, shrank from any effort to shake or change the faith of others" (qtd. in Tóibín 14). Gregory "looked now for poetry and romance" from "stone-breakers and potato-diggers and paupers in the workhouse and beggars at my own door" (qtd. in Tóibín 36). Rather than attempting to convert peoples' religion, Gregory turned to restoring respect for the peasantry and Irish folklore and converted any negative opinions of them.

If Gregory did participate in the Persse family practice of going from house-to-house, with the ulterior motive of trying to convert people to Protestantism, then she later left it in the past and changed her reason for travelling from door to door. Her folklore-collecting practice healed the previous associations attached to her neighbourhood rounds. At the early stages of her conversion, Irish folklore was an anaesthetic that numbed her fractious past. By 1902, however, it was a transplant that restored Gregory as well as Ireland; it was a metaphorical panacea that Gregory had mixed together for her own healing. She desired to excise both the denotations and connotations that came with the English-speaking and Anglo-Irish colonial class. Rather than dispense Protestantism she would gather to herself; she would collect. She wished to be converted.

* * *

Both Gregory and Cathleen Ni Houlihan begin again and, somatically, the eponymous play is connected to Gregory's life. Hynes's directorial decision to make Cathleen look as much like Gregory as possible revives a stratum of the play that has been buried under the legend of Maud Gonne's 1902 performance. It is interesting that Gregory played this part herself in three theatre performances beginning "[o]n March 18, 1919, three days after her sixty-seventh birthday" because "actress Mary Walker [a name later changed to Máire Nic Shiubhlaigh] could not get to Dublin in time for a scheduled performance of *Cathleen Ni Houlihan*" (Kohfeldt 259). According to Walker, the actress who was also an Irish republican, Gregory "often spoke of the occasion afterwards, referring proudly and a trifle pathetically to her appearance in the play as the realisation of a life-long ambition" (*The Splendid Years* 30).[21] In a journal entry, Gregory posed a rhetorical question in parenthesis: "(after all what is wanted but a hag and a voice?)" (*Lady Gregory's Journals* 56).[22] Kohfeldt writes, "[S]he

[21] For more information about Gregory's performance, see Caehlin O'Malley Bell's *Being Ireland: Lady Gregory in Cathleen Ni Houlihan* (2008).

[22] Gregory is also quoted in Kohfeldt's *Lady Gregory: The Woman Behind the Irish Renaissance*: "After all, what is wanted but a hag and a voice?" (259).

played the old woman who turns out to be a 'young girl with the walk of a queen' whom she and Willie had created together fifteen years before, and who in some ways epitomized her own metamorphosis from obscure widow to guiding spirit of the Irish Renaissance" (259).[23] However, it is more likely that Gregory chose Cathleen Ni Houlihan to be a role model for her life, so much so that she perhaps based the character on herself or, rather, who she wanted to become. To Gregory, the role was simply "a hag and a voice," and it was her job to bring the rest.

A Yeats-Gregory collaboration, this one-act play is set in the "[*i*]*nterior of a cottage close to Killala*" in County Mayo in 1798, the year when French soldiers allied with Irish rebels in order to overthrow the oppressive British rule (*VPl* 214).[24] It is the eve of the character Michael Gillane's wedding when a "Poor Old Woman" arrives at the cottage and then later metamorphoses into "a young girl" that "had the walk of a queen" (lines 277, 347–48; act 1). This *cailleach* has two main aims: "The hope of getting my beautiful fields back again; the hope of putting the strangers out of my house" (lines 252–54). She has "good friends," the French soldiers, who "are gathering to help me now," and she "must call the [Irish]

[23]There is a photograph, which captures "Augusta Gregory in the role of Cathleen ni Houlihan," that was taken by an unknown photographer on 21 March 1919 ("Playing Cathleen ni Houlihan"; New York Public Library; courtesy of Colin Smythe). The New York Public Library (NYPL) state that this photograph, which is "[c]ourtesy of Colin Smythe," was captured when "[t]wo journalists came to the theater during rehearsal on March 21, 1919 and took this photograph of her on stage with Arthur Shields, who played the role of Michael Gillane, the young man Cathleen inspires to follow her and fight for Ireland" ("Playing Cathleen ni Houlihan"). The New York Public Library add that "Shields had fought in the Easter Rising of 1916" ("Playing Cathleen ni Houlihan"). In a typed journal entry, dated March 1919, Gregory wrote that "my face was painted with grease paint—white with black under the eyes and red inside the lids—dreadful!" and that "[l]uckily, my own hair is grey enough without a wig" ("Lady Gregory as Cathleen ni Houlihan"; *Lady Gregory's Journals* 56). Gregory grew into the role with each performance. Based on her journal entry, the New York Public Library informs, "[a]t the first performance, she was 'a little hoarse and felt miserable' but 'got through all right,' and then grew in confidence in her remaining appearances" ("Playing Cathleen ni Houlihan"; *Lady Gregory's Journals* 56-57). Although she was "a little hoarse and felt miserable" on her first production (18 March 1919) due to "a slight cold" and was "shock[ed] to find the auditorium was black darkness" so that she "thought for a moment the curtain was still down and hesitated," she was "even more nervous than the first night but got through without prompts and had my own two curtains" on the second performance on 19 March 1919 (*Lady Gregory's Journals* 56–57). By the third performance on 20 March 1919, Gregory "played the part better and with more confidence than before" (*Lady Gregory's Journals* 58).

[24]The quotations for *Cathleen Ni Houlihan* (1902) are taken from *The Variorum Edition of the Plays of W. B. Yeats* (1966), edited by Russell K. Alspach.

neighbours together to welcome them" (lines 256–57, 261–62). This echoes Gregory's practice of calling upon the neighbours to gather folklore from them, thus recruiting them as preservers of Irish literature.

Cathleen Ni Houlihan starts out as an old woman and, after fomenting rebellion, is reborn, young, and enamoured with nationalism. At the resolution, Michael Gillane leaves his fiancée, a good home, money, and "grand clothes" in order to fight for Ireland's independence (line 12). The performance of the play in April 1902 in St. Teresa's Hall on Clarendon Street, staged by the same company that would later be called the Abbey Theatre, had negative health implications in terms of violent public reactions. However, Gregory did not advocate violence. In an article, "The Felons of Our Land" (1900), Gregory realised how much she had changed and specified that "[j]ust now … I seem possessed with the passion for Ireland, for my country," but she made it clear that she "will not take a life" (qtd. in Pethica, "'Our Kathleen'" 216; ellipsis in source). *Cathleen Ni Houlihan* was traditionally seen as a dangerous play, as evidenced by Stephen Gwynn, a critic who questioned "if such plays should be produced unless one was prepared for people to go out to shoot and be shot" (qtd. in Tóibín 47–48). Whilst simultaneously colonising the play by claiming it as his own in the late poem, "The Man and the Echo" (1939), Yeats asked, "Did that play of mine send out / Certain men the English shot?" (*VP* lines 11–12; *Last Poems*). This self-castigation misses something crucial that comes to light if we switch our focus from Yeats to Gregory: that rebirth and change, and not just bloodshed, are central to the play.

Following this, Cathleen Ni Houlihan can be interpreted as a spiritual character, who is reborn as a young person. Peter, Patrick Gillane's father, poses an interrogative: "Did you see an old woman going down the path?" (lines 345–46). His son, Patrick, replies with an assertion: "I did not, but I saw a young girl, and she had the walk of a queen" (lines 347–48). This question-and-answer sequence forms the final two lines of the play, and it provides an answer for Gregory because her new identity is the "young" Irish nationalist with "the walk of a queen." James Pethica analyses Gregory's early draft of *Cathleen Ni Houlihan*, which is held in the Berg Collection at the New York Public Library ("'Our Kathleen'" 210–11). According to Pethica, Gregory writes, "'All this mine alone,' at the end of the first section of ten pages, and 'This with W. B. Y.' at the head of the second section," which meet "at a point just after the Old Woman enters the Gillane cottage" (210–11). Pethica argues, "The satisfied tone apparent in 'All this mine alone' is particularly suggestive of recent accomplishment, and Lady Gregory would have been less likely to note her personal share in the work so self-consciously once close collaboration with Yeats had become relatively routine for her" (211). Gregory herself "recalled having written 'all but all of' *Cathleen Ni Houlihan*" in a journal entry in 1922, which points to the centrality of her ideas in this play (qtd. in Pethica 207). Though critical opinions about the proportion of the play that can be attributed to each of its authors vary, it is evident that it carries the stamp of both.[25] The transformation that Cathleen Ni Houlihan undergoes from aged woman to rejuvenated nationalist avatar, though, at least carries the intriguing possibility that she is a dramatic doppelgänger for Gregory herself.

The muse that inspired this play appeared in a distinctively Irish form. The vision for *Cathleen Ni Houlihan* appeared to Yeats, in his own account, not from literary beginnings, but in his own personal aisling. In a letter to Gregory, in February 1903, Yeats wrote:

> One night I had a dream almost as distinct as a vision, of a cottage where there was well-being and firelight and talk of a marriage, and into the midst of that cottage there came an old woman in a long cloak. She was Ireland herself, that Cathleen ni Houlihan for whom so many songs have been sung and about whom so many stories have been told ... I thought if I could write this out as a little play I could make others see my dream as I had seen it, but I could not get down out of that high window of dramatic verse, and in spite of all you had done for me I had not the country speech. One has to live among the people, like you, ... before one can think the thoughts of the people and speak with their tongue. We turned my dream into the little play, "Cathleen ni Hoolihan," and when we gave it to the little theatre in Dublin and found that the working people liked it, you helped me to put my other dramatic fables into speech. (*CL* 3: 321–22)

[25] For a counterview to Pethica's argument, which downplays Gregory's contribution to *Cathleen Ni Houlihan*, see Aisling Carlin's journal article titled "To 'make others see my dream as I had seen it': Yeats's aesthetics in *Cathleen Ni Houlihan*" (2013). Whilst Pethica's argument, in Carlin's words, is for "Lady Gregory's role as at least co-author, if not primary author, on this occasion," Carlin counter-argues that "the complexity of structure and detail justifies Yeats's authorship of the play" and seeks to "further prove Yeats's justification in taking *Cathleen ni Houlihan* as primarily his creation, notwithstanding Lady Gregory's collaboration" (65, 76, 67).

Yeats's words reveal his sense of his inability (at this point in his career) to produce the kind of "naturalist" dialogue that dominates the play. Yeats is always ambivalent about Henrik Ibsen, a Norwegian playwright who is often called "the father of realism": his cultural nationalism (and anti-colonialism) is admired by Yeats, but not his naturalist dramaturgy, which Yeats (unlike Gregory and Martyn) did not find congenial. Hence the strangeness of *Cathleen Ni Houlihan*: it is a naturalist play (dominated by economic issues) which concludes by rejecting not only materialism but also naturalism, in the symbolic transformation of the title character. Bernard O'Donoghue defines an aisling as "a vision poem in which a woman representing Ireland appears to the dreaming narrator and offers some insight or prophecy, usually about the fate of Ireland" (420). This poetic form contributed to preserving Irish because it "served as a claim for a cultural distinction—the sophistication of Bardic poetry—at a time when Irish was failing as a written language" (O'Donoghue 432). Traditionally, "the narrator of the poem falls asleep, usually in a gloomy frame of mind prompted by poverty or political circumstances, and is visited by a visionary woman of great beauty (though sometimes old, weary, and withered: hence the brilliance of the reversal of the theme at the end of Yeats/Gregory's *Cathleen Ni Houlihan*)" (O'Donoghue 421). However, Cathleen Ni Houlihan's role as a physical embodiment of the aisling itself has so far been overlooked in academic criticism.[26] Cathleen is an awake and conscious form of an aisling because she predicts the "pale cheeks" and declining health of the Irish people (line 310). She then induces a delayed dreamlike state upon Michael, who has "the look of a man that has got the touch," admits he had "forgotten" about his wedding, and "doesn't hear a word" that his family are "saying" to him (lines 317–18, 328, 339). Yeats had dreamt about a *cailleach*, a legendary female figure from early Irish mythology that manifests in two main forms: an old and a young woman.

In early Irish tradition, the *cailleach* figure in general is explicitly a nationalism of guise, and there are two main guises: young and old. In *The Cold of May Day Monday: An Approach to Irish Literature* (2014), Robert Welch provides a comprehensive history of the folk tradition, which is useful for tracking original sources that contain the *cailleach* and her double form. The *cailleach* has one of her earliest written incarnations in "The Hag of Beare," an anonymous Irish poem about an elderly woman

[26] It is a surprising omission from Robert Welch's book.

remembering her youth, written in around the tenth century, and then later translated by Gregory in *The Kiltartan Poetry Book: Prose Translations from the Irish* (1919). The seventeenth-century-born Munster poet Egan O'Rahilly's "Gile an Gile" ("Brightness of Brightness") is a vision poem that was likely to have been composed in the early eighteenth century, which tells the tale of a beautiful woman that represents Ireland and is awaiting freedom (*Poems of Egan O'Rahilly* 18–21). Hedge schoolteacher Brian Merriman wrote "Cúirt an Mheán Oíche" ("The Midnight Court") around the time of 1780, and it is "the last major Gaelic poem before the revival of Irish in the twentieth century" (Welch 88)[27]:

> The poem opens in the aisling format, that convention where the poet falls asleep in the countryside and is granted a vision of Ireland in female form, who looks forward to the return of the Stuart and her freedom from the bondage she has to endure from the stranger, England. The aisling form is connected to the legends associated with the tutelary goddesses, the sovereignty archetype, and the Hag, who, as in the stories of the Hag of Beare, can be both young and old, beautiful and horrifying, and also capable of shifting between these manifestations. (Welch 88)

Welch proposes that "after Merriman, while the Gaelic literary tradition in its formal manifestation went into decline, there began to develop, based on cultural strata that had been in existence for over a thousand years, a folk and oral tradition of truly impressive range and sophistication" (91). He states that "[i]t seems as if Irish literary and linguistic culture has the capacity, at times of dereliction and decline, to find new modes of expression, where the ancient energies get rechannelled into different directions and new forms" (Welch 91–92). In reference to later years, Welch writes that "[t]he effect the recovery of folklore had on Irish literature in the latter part of the nineteenth century was to compel many writers and artists into a deep examination of questions of identity" as "Yeats, Lady Gregory, Joseph Campbell, and many others discovered, among the Irish country people, stories and poems that seemed to bring them into a living relationship with some of the deepest strata of European culture itself" (98). The two versions of the hag that appear in *Cathleen Ni Houlihan* are rooted in the myths of the *cailleach*.

[27] *Cúirt an Mheán Oíche* is a comedy and a satire as well as an aisling.

It is possible that Gregory's and Yeats's discovery of the *cailleach* and its many forms was a gradual process. When Yeats's younger brother Robert died, he experienced the "realization of death" as "I heard people telling how my mother and the servant had heard the banshee crying the night before he died" (*Autobiographies* 55; *Reveries Over Childhood and Youth*). Ó Crualaoich confirms that the *cailleach* figure inspired the "services" of the *bean sí* or banshee or keener (29). In her book, *Celtic Ireland* (1889), Sophie Bryant states, "The ben-sidhe, pronounced *banshee*, has descended to our times, as the guardian spirit of certain Irish families, which manifests itself in some way when a death is at hand" (101). Yeats's early exposure to one aspect of the *cailleach* form was followed by his interest in "a wise woman that lived in Clare some years ago," known as Biddy Early, whose memory he discovered on one of his folklore-collecting walks in Coole in 1896 (*Mythologies* 14). This would be an encounter with healing and the *bean feasa* (wise woman figure), which was another strand of the *cailleach* tradition.

There were readings about witches that were available to Gregory and Yeats, though these were about witches and not the *cailleach* specifically.[28] For example, Gregory owned Lady Jane Wilde's *Poems by Speranza* (1864), some of which poems included witches. When Yeats wrote *Stories of the Red Hanrahan* (1897), a short collection of stories told using the eponymous fictional character, he included a poem about "Cathleen, the daughter of Houlihan" in which he misspells *Cailleach na Béara* as "Clooth-na-Bare" (*Mythologies* 155). This same mis-transliteration occurs in Yeats's note to "The Hosting of the Sidhe," a poem in which a group of mythological Irish characters (notably Caoilte and Niamh) are "riding from Knocknarea/And over the grave of Clooth-na-Bare," from the 1899 collection titled *The Wind Among the Reeds* (*VP* lines 1–2). Similar to the "pale cheeks" that are mentioned in *Cathleen Ni Houlihan*, Caoilte and Niamh sing a song within the poem "The Hosting of the Sidhe" that begins by saying that "*Our cheeks are pale*," which suggests that Yeats perhaps drew upon this poem when writing Cathleen's monologue (*VPl* line 310; *VP* line 7). There, in *The Wind Among the Reeds*, Yeats writes, "Clooth-na-Bare would mean the old woman of Bare, but is evidently a

[28] Yeats owned Edwin Sidney Hartland's *Mythology and Folktales: Their Relations and Interpretation* (1900), Joseph Ennemosier's two-volumed *The History of Magic* (1854), and Walter Yeeling Evans Wentz's PhD thesis titled *The Fairy-Faith in Celtic Countries* (1909) (O'Shea 118, 91, 299).

corruption of Cailleac Bare" (*VP* 802). This would suggest that by (at the latest) 1899, Yeats is aware of the "corruption," but he chooses to keep it—presumably for metrical and euphonious reasons. This spelling mistake is picked up in poet Thomas MacDonagh's *Literature in Ireland* (1916), a book in Gregory's library (*Catalogue* 39). MacDonagh writes that "nothing is gained, surely, by that extraordinary perversion of the Irish name of the Old Woman of Beare, *Cailleach na Béara*" and adds that "[t]he word *clooth* is not Irish; it has no meaning" (51). This misspelling could suggest that Yeats's knowledge of the *cailleach* was still in process. Both Yeats and Gregory perhaps helped each other to deepen their knowledge about the *cailleach* over the years.

Ó Crualaoich argues that "the services of the *bean ghlúine* (midwife), the *bean feasa* (wise-woman) and the *bean chaointe* (keening-woman)" were "three human female personae whose *cailleach*-inspired (and derived) performance of service to the community was so essential" (29). They were known "to diagnose and minister to the stricken individual and the stricken community" (Ó Crualaoich 72). Their "female roles were activated at times of life-crisis in what was a predominantly patriarchal society, as a coping mechanism in the face of the trauma of major life transitions and afflictions" (72). These "serviceable coping mechanisms" are "of a ritual and psychotherapeutic sort" and occur "at times of individual and group affliction" (11). This brings to mind Gregory's services to her neighbourhood, which involved dispensing medicine and dyeing flannel, at a time when both her and Ireland were undergoing a major transformation. Ó Crualaoich proposes that "the Irish wise-woman is a healer – by predominantly symbolic means – of crisis trauma" as "the roles of midwife and keener focus on the life traumas of birthing and dying" and "that of the *bean feasa* focuses on the affliction traumas" related to "health or property" (72–73). Ó Crualaoich postulates that "the many legends of the resort to the wise-woman and of her prescience, may be regarded as a form of traditional, 'therapy' that exhibits features comparable to the professional psychotherapy practiced today" (12). For instance, the "flesh-and-blood, *bean chaointe* (the keening-woman at the wake), reveals how such a 'real' woman can be a manifestation of mythological meanings and values" in terms of "the service of emotional well-being" (Ó Crualaoich 11–12). Ó Crualaoich's illumination of the role of *cailleach* as outlet for emotion and healer draws attention to an aspect of Cathleen Ni Houlihan that is less discussed than her role as a catalyst for violence.

Cathleen Ni Houlihan represents a form of self-invention for Gregory. This protagonist goes into the play an old crone; she comes out rejuvenated as "a young girl" with "the walk of a queen" (lines 347–48). Gregory's self-invention began when she was about forty; she achieves renewal by 1902, with the publication of *Cuchulain of Muirthemne*. Many scholars have pointed out that the play shows the *cailleach* in her two traditional guises (old and young) and indeed it does. However, the play offers a spiritual portrait of the progress made by Gregory herself. She reinvented her own life and underwent a period of revival, recovery, and restoration from 1892 to 1902. Her husband and Governor of Ceylon, William Gregory, died in March 1892; this also marked the death of her English imperialistic beliefs. In her reidentification process, Gregory's progress seems partly guided by the examples of both Biddy Early and Cathleen Ni Houlihan.

The revival of health in *Cathleen Ni Houlihan* is associated with the loss of health and of everything else in life so that the nation might be revived. The breakdown of health and the loss of strength is foreshadowed in Cathleen Ni Houlihan's requirement for recruitment: "If any one would give me help he must give me himself, he must give me all" (lines 243–44). This suggests that the Irish Revival is for the nation, not the individual. This utilitarian approach is epitomised when the old woman reveals that the opposite of restoration seems to be happening in order to restore the health of Ireland and the many, where life is damaged and destroyed before revival can take place:

> It is a hard service they take that help me.
> Many that are red-cheeked now will be pale-cheeked;
> many that have been free to walk the hills and the
> bogs and the rushes will be sent to walk hard streets
> in far countries; many a good plan will be broken;
> many that have gathered money will not stay to
> spend it; many a child will be born and there will be
> no father at its christening to give it a name. They
> that have red cheeks will have pale cheeks for my
> sake, and for all that, they will think they are well
> paid. (lines 302–12)

These anti-medical aspects are significant because this play is reminiscent of the journey to the Tír na nÓg, where youth comes at a horrific cost to mortals. Cathleen becomes young again, but the people transmute from being "red-cheeked" and become "pale-cheeked" as a result, and health is lost for this cause.

There is a parasitic effect on life—something gothic and vampirical enters the scene. R. F. Foster has discussed this trope in Anglo-Irish literature, amongst other scholars, and interprets Bram Stoker's *Dracula* (1897) as an Anglo-Irish parable.[29] Confirming Yeats's knowledge of vampires, Foster informs, "Yeats knew Stoker; he inscribed a copy of *The Countess Kathleen* to him in 1892, read *Dracula* with Ezra Pound, and was only put off a proposed visit to Dracula's original castle (though Yeats thought it was in Austria, not Transylvania) by the outbreak of a world war in 1914" ("Protestant Magic" 252; Longenbach 108–09). Bruce Stewart poses a question: "How far is Bram Stoker's *Dracula* (1897) an Irish novel?" (238). He adds, "To this question Irish critics have recently supplied dramatic answers arising from the resemblance between the blood-sucking aristocrat and the economic practices of the Anglo-Irish gentry" and responds, "Not only is it unlikely that Count Dracula was inscribed as a portrait of the rapacious landlord of popular memory, it is more probable that the vampiric tendencies of the villain were designed to represent the kind of atavistic violence commonly attributed by members of Stoker's class to Land League activists and, by implication, to Charles Stewart Parnell — whom they regarded as puppet-master of the agrarian agitators" (Stewart 239; Moses 68). Stewart argues, "It may be best, therefore, to suppose that Dracula represents *both* the landlord *and* the forces behind agrarian crime in the Land War era" (243). Stewart selects references from the Irish revolutionary James Fintan Lalor's contributions to *The Irish Felon* (1848), a nationalist journal that the British government discontinued after five issues, "that might be applied with little alteration to a clique of aristocratic vampires" (241). For example, Lalor comments, "Strangers they are in this land they call theirs — strangers here and strangers everywhere, owning no country and owned by none; rejecting Ireland, and rejected by England" (qtd. in Stewart 241). Gregory and Yeats perhaps embodied this idea in Cathleen Ni Houlihan's "hope of putting the strangers out of my house" (lines 253–54). Cathleen is the opposite: she

[29] Read R. F. Foster's "Protestant Magic: W. B. Yeats and the Spell of Irish History" (1989), Bruce Stewart's "Bram Stoker's *Dracula*: Possessed by the Spirit of the Nation?" (1999), and Matthew Gibson's "Bram Stoker and the Treaty of Berlin (1878)" (2004).

will destroy and damage, suck the lifeblood, turn red cheeks to pale, but she will do so *for* Ireland.

Cathleen Ni Houlihan's type one conditional sentence is paramount: "If they are put down to-day they will get the upper hand to-morrow" (lines 258–59). After this hypothetical sentence, a stage direction informs that "[*She gets up*]" (line 259). This paralinguistic feature indicates that the personified Ireland is "*get*[*ting*] *up*" and rising in strength due to the Irish peoples' sacrifices. The sacrifice of health is an interesting trope as, ironically, the play itself cured and healed and created a blank slate that sought to restore Ireland to perfect health and restore Gregory's life as an individual. The old woman sings:

> They shall be remembered for ever,
> They shall be alive for ever,
> They shall be speaking for ever,
> The people shall hear them for ever. (lines 313–16)

The people who offered up their health for the national cause live forever in the Irish and international memory. The anaphora is significant as the third person pronoun "[t]hey" becomes "[t]he people" in the final line, implicating that the individuals are given up for the collective nation. Every line of the song ends on "for ever" and serves as a ploce that evokes the immortality of this sacrifice.

* * *

Gregory's later sole-authored play *The Golden Apple: A Play for Kiltartan Children* (1916) shows a preoccupation with ageing and death and the possibility of renewal. It could be argued that there is degree to which the herbal lore in this play is "window dressing," there to give the play the feel of a wonder tale through including characters such as witches and giants. The specific and undeniable links to traditional medicine in the play that are also present in Gregory's folk medical texts, however, shows that her herbal knowledge even reached a play for which the intended audiences are children. In this play, written for youth living in the nearby Kiltartan parish in County Galway, the King of Ireland is ill and beyond the healing of the royal doctor. There is a treatment, however, in "the Garden at the

World's End" (275; act 3, sc. 2).[30] It takes the form of "the golden apple that will cure any sickness at all or any wound" (216; act 1, sc. 1). The healing apple is the crux for an exploration of medical cures, health metaphors, and the elixir of life. As such, it shows the preoccupations with regeneration and renewal that are such a central part of *Cathleen* stayed with her as her life continued.

Rury, the King's son, journeys to find this apple with his steward and encounters a witch and a match-maker giant (named Fatach Mor) along the way. The giant's wife gives Rury an enchanted "ball of flax" that is "[t]wisted ... on a crooked holly stick" that has "a charm" to "bring you through all the world" (238; act 1, sc. 4). Rury takes the apple and falls in love with the King of Spain's daughter, Muireann, whom the witch has entrapped in the garden. Meanwhile, the giant consults the doctor about symptoms including fatigue, loss of appetite, and feeling "sickly," but he receives a false diagnosis (248; act 2, sc. 2). The doctor steals the apple so that he can present it to the King himself; the apple holds the elixir of life as, on eating it, the King, like Cathleen in the earlier play, went "backward in age" and "look[ed] elegant in the face" (275; act 3, sc. 2).

Gregory gleaned much of her information about apples and medicine from her earlier mythological works, in which this fruit is employed to heal warriors and extend life. In "The Sons of Tuireann," the second chapter in *Gods and Fighting Men* (1904), there are "three apples ... from the Garden in the East of the World" that "do not leave the pain of wounds or the vexation of sickness on any one that eats them, and they do not lessen by being eaten for ever" (33).[31] Gregory, in *The Kiltartan Poetry Book* (1919), associates apples with the Tír na nÓg: "In ancient times the poets told of this Country of the Young, with its trees bearing fruit and blossom at the one time; its golden apples that gave lasting life" (14). Yeats draws upon

[30] Unless otherwise declared, all quotations for Gregory's plays are taken from *Selected Plays of Lady Gregory* (1983), edited by Mary FitzGerald.

[31] When the giant's wife states that "[t]here is some doctors who can recognise what sickness is on a man by the smoke they see going out of the chimney of his house," this is a cross-reference to medical information in *Cuchulain of Muirthemne*: "Now, Fingan was the greatest physician in all Ireland, and it was said of him that he could tell what a person's sickness was by looking at the smoke of the house he was in" (*Golden Apple* 249-50; *Cuchulain of Muirthemne* 246). In *The Golden Apple*, the doctor diagnoses the giant with having "swallowed a water-worm or an eel" (250). This is inspired by Gregory's "Herb Healing" chapter in *Poets and Dreamers* (1903), where she writes about a person who was "feeling a worm in [their] side that is as big as an eel"; one of the cures that they tried involved "put[ting] sea-grass to it" (118–19).

"[t]he golden apples of the sun" in "The Song of Wandering Aengus" (1899), a mythological poem about *Aengus Óg* ("Young Aengus") being "old with wandering" (lines 24, 17). The golden apple being associated with rejuvenation suggests the promise of a new life for the "old" protagonist of "Wandering Aengus" (line 17). The end of the poem suggests that he might never actually find those apples, just as he may never ever catch that "glimmering girl," and that is the pathos and beauty of the poem (line 13). There is a reversal of Christian mythology, and it was pagan Ireland versus the Christian worldview of original sin, the apple, suffering, and death. Gregory restored the apple, a theologically fallen fruit that humanity misused in the Garden of Eden in Genesis, as a healing food "that will cure any sickness at all or any wound" in *The Golden Apple* (216). Gregory, by extension, sought to restore Ireland as well as other countries that had also suffered from colonial mistreatment, and replant them into a peaceful garden that provides a new space for universal growth and healing. In *The Schools' Manuscript Collection* (*NFCS*), students across the Republic of Ireland gathered folklore for the *National Folklore Collection* (*NFC*) from their neighbours and family members in the 1930s. An anonymous teacher told collector Mary Kennedy a story titled "The Magic Apples," in which "[t]he King of Ireland" sends "three brothers" to collect "magic apples growing in a garden in Hesbernia" (126).[32] "Hesbernia" sounds like "Hibernia," which is the classical Latinate word for "Ireland." If "Hibernia" is the intended word, the Tír na nÓg and the mythical apples can be traced back to Gregory's homeland.

As well as being credited with powers of rejuvenation and healing in mythology, apples were credited with salutary power in the Irish countryside. They were an ingredient that Early sought in order to cure myriad illnesses. In Meda Ryan's *Biddy Early: The Wise Woman of Clare* (1978), informant Dolly Steward attests, "Nettles, potatoes, apples, honey, all these things were plentiful and could be used as cures for all kinds of ailments" (34). In both of those sources of Revival literature, mythology, and folk belief, apples shine.

[32] *NFCS* 0904: 126; teacher; Collector: Mary Kennedy, Baile Uí Mhurchadha, Borris, Ballymurphy, County Carlow, October 1937-December 1938. Teacher: Michael Ó Seachnasaigh. In this source, the following authorial information is also written: "Told by our teacher who heard it from Martin Dalton of Ballyine, Borris, about 50 years ago. He was then about 45 years of age." This shows that this story was circulating in Ireland in Gregory's lifetime.

At the exposition, the witch and the gardener engage in a discussion about replanting "the little Tree of Power" that holds the "*one golden apple*" (215; act 1, sc. 1). This tree is "used to the country of the sun" (216; act 1, sc. 1). The gardener advises the witch against "rising the roots" as, like Gregory's walled garden at Coole, the walls provide "good shelter" for "the little tree" (216; act 1, sc. 1). It is interesting that the gardener's reasoning as to why the tree should not be uprooted is hinged on March, a month that was an important milestone in Gregory's life.

March was a pivotal month in Gregory's personal revival process. The gardener instructs the witch to "[w]ait till the month of March comes at it and you'll see it's a great persecuting it will get, and it not to be minded the way it is" (216; act 1, sc. 1). Addressing Rury, Simon says, "What ails you to be in such a hurry! Is it that the King gave you for a mother the wind of March?" (256; act 2, sc. 3). Gregory built her own shelter with an anti-imperial identity so that, when she was susceptible to the personal events and harsh elements that occurred in multiple March months, she would not be "persecute[ed]" but liberated through not being "minded" or shaken in her new selfhood. Kohfeldt notes, "Dying on March 22, her mother added another date to Augusta's month of anniversaries, which already contained her birthday, her wedding day, and the day of Sir William's death" (102). Gregory revealed that the deaths of her mother (Frances Persse) in March 1896 and her eldest sister (Elizabeth Shawe-Taylor) in August 1896 caused "a strange blank" that unleashed a "sense of my foundations having slipped away" (qtd. in Kohfeldt 103). It is fascinating that her familial and marital ends are marked by March, a month that signifies the closure of winter and the beginning of spring; March 1896 held Gregory's *re-birth*day, which was the fourth anniversary of her husband's death, when she was reborn as new woman who would grow to become an anti-imperialist.

Throughout the play, there are references to the witch's practice of travelling from door to door and begging. Pampogue, the witch's daughter, asks early in Act One Scene One if she can accompany her mother on these outings because "I would like well to travel among neighbours and to go visiting at country houses by the roadside" and she insists that "[i]t is time for me to be giving out food to company and keeping the keys of a house" (217; act 1, sc. 1). She accuses, "You yourself go out gathering news or making news far and wide" and suggests, "It would be more fitting I to be doing that, and you that are up in age to be sitting spinning at the wheel" (217; act 1, sc. 1). Pampogue accuses her mother of dismissing

Rury later in the final act and, perplexed by her lack of freedom, tells her that "you have the world to ramble, begging from door to door!" (273; act 3, sc. 1). Indeed, after the apple is stolen from them, the King's son and the steward are at one point "begging on the road" (277; act 3, sc. 2). The stories that Gregory recorded in *Visions and Beliefs in the West of Ireland* (1920) either depict old women as healers, or as having powers that could cast misfortune upon whole households and livestock, a belief perhaps reflected in Michael's aversion to strangers in *Cathleen Ni Houlihan*: "I'd sooner a stranger not to come to the house the night before my wedding" (2: 20, 123, 230–31; *VPl* lines 133–35). Gregory was aware of the fear that surrounded old women who begged from home-to-home in the Irish countryside. Through giving the shape-shifting witch the sinister role of moving from house-to-house, Gregory also exerts disapproval of proselytising and aims to plaster over this fractious history by metamorphosing her own local travels into a folklore-collecting mission. Gregory casts a negative character to fulfil this role, which suggests that she had her own doubts about its ethics.

Clothes play a crucial role in *The Golden Apple*, *Cathleen Ni Houlihan*, and in Gregory's neighbourhood duties. In *The Golden Apple*, Muireann is forced "to shape and to sew a dress for Pampogue" (219; act 1, sc. 1). This wedding dress is never worn as Rury does not marry Pampogue regardless of her "riches" and "estate," and it is Muireann who ends up "*wearing … fine clothes*" (271; act 3, sc. 1; 280; act 3, sc. 1). In *Cathleen Ni Houlihan*, Bridget's "*examining* [*of*] *the clothes, pulling the seams and trying the lining of the pockets*" at the exposition is similarly futile (line 47). This is because Michael is later torn between "*look*[*ing*] *at the clothes and turn*[*ing*] *towards the inner room*" and "*the sound of the cheering outside*" that makes him "*stop*" at the resolution (line 328). When "[*t*]*he clothes slip from Michael's arm*," Gregory completes a cyclical structure that shows Michael leaving materialism to follow the spiritual Cathleen Ni Houlihan and therefore Ireland (line 332). This is formally reiterated or reinforced in the play's repudiation of Ibsenite naturalism in its symbolic close: this too marks a dramaturgical shift from materialism to idealism. As there is a link between the theme of materialism and the literal clothing materials, there is a materialism and material pun at work in *Cathleen Ni Houlihan*.

By including remedies in *The Golden Apple*, Gregory relates the world of medicine and healing to the Irish Revival, a literary movement that involved medical metaphors about physical health and bodily cures. In the play, Simon takes the "hot stones on the hearth" and "put them to [the King's] feet" (224; act 1, sc. 2). Whereas, the doctor takes "[t]he skin of a sheep that is after being killed, fresh and warm" and "wrap[s] it about his body" in the hope that it "might put some heat into his blood" (223; act 1, sc. 2).[33] The King, however, is unhappy with the sheepskin and instead asks the doctor a question: "Had you no lion from the Eastern World to go skin, ...?" (225; act 1, sc. 2). Here, literature about folk medicine can help us to understand these developments. Lady Jane Wilde's first volume of *Ancient Legends, Mystic Charms, and Superstitions of Ireland* (1887) provides information about these healing methods.

Simon's preferred therapy, the hot stones, is an ancient practice in both Ireland and India that is "the most effective cure known for pains in the bones and feverish disorders" (Wilde 245). Although "*[h]e brings stones and puts them at end of bed*," the usual method involves a stone bath that is "covered over with branches" and "hot water is then poured on the stones, and the patient crouches over the heated vapour evolved until a violent perspiration is produced, which carries off the disease, or the pains in the members, without fail" (224: act 1, sc. 2; Wilde 1: 245). Wilde notes that "[t]he sweating bath of the Irish was made quite on the same principles" as the Indian version, and she compliments women of all nationalities on their medical prowess as "amongst all primitive tribes and nations, women have always shown the highest skill in the treatment of disease, and have been rightly accounted the best doctors, and the most learned in mystic medicinal lore" (Wilde 1: 245, 244). In particular, Wilde congratulates "old women" that "display wonderful knowledge of the mystic nature and power of herbs, and are most expert in the cure of disease" (1: 244). It is interesting that Lady Wilde's text seeks to validate Indian and Irish remedies and to valorise the folk knowledge circulated among women. In both national and gender terms, the medical was the political.

The sheep skin, the royal doctor's recommendation in Gregory's *The Golden Apple*, has a concomitant in Lady Jane Wilde's story: "The Fenian Knights: A Legend of the West." In this, the legendary Fionn mac Cumhaill foresees a dangerous warrior approaching the Fenians and a comrade is later injured in battle as "the skin of his thighs" is lost (*Ancient Legends* 1: 159). The Fenian cure is akin to the doctor's treatment in Gregory's play as "[t]hen they killed a sheep, and wrapped the fleece

[33] This is reminiscent of "the pig skin of Tuis, King of Greece" that "heals all the wounds and all the sickness of the world" in "The Sons of Tuireann" in *Gods and Fighting Men* (1904) (Gregory 33).

round him warm from the animal to heal him" and "[s]o he was cured, but ever after, strange to relate, seven stone of wool were annually shorn from his body as long as he lived" (1: 159). These two medical approaches, the hot stones and the sheep skin, come from the mouths of two differently qualified people and both practices are equally valid. There is a doctor in the play, but he does not have a monopoly on medical knowledge. Folk knowledge had a role to play in healing in the world of *The Golden Apple*. Gregory is possibly breaking down the barriers of medical practitioners suggesting that, at the time, ordinary people were just as entitled to maintaining health as qualified doctors.

Gregory showed much interest in medicine within Fenian legends, which is illuminated in *Gods and Fighting Men* (1904), a chrestomathy of ancient Irish sagas. In "The Hunt of Slieve Cuilinn," a tale within this work, a *cailleach* who is "a woman of the Sidhe, Miluchradh, daughter of Cuilinn" is presented as a "young girl" who "seemed to be some way sorrowful and downhearted" (Gregory 309, 306, 307). She lures Finn into a lake to retrieve her ring, which transforms him into "an ailing, downhearted old man, without leaping, without running, without walk, grey and sorrowful" (Gregory 308). This echoes Yeats's resolution to *The Wanderings of Oisin* (1889), when Oisin is left "[w]ithout laughter, a show unto children, alone with remembrance and fear" and is "[a]ll emptied of purple hours as a beggar's cloak in the rain" (*VPl* lines 218–19). Gregory also brings this polysyndetic listing into *The Golden Apple* when the doctor asks the giant a question: "Do you go walking or leaping or running, for to give exercise to your limbs?" (248; act 2, sc. 2). Oisin remaining young and Cathleen Ni Houlihan being reborn and Finn regaining his youth are key storylines that explore the central themes of fear and old age.

In "The Hunt of Slieve Cuilinn," the Fianna "gave three loud sorrowful cries" when they realise that the "old man" is Finn and "Conan of the sharp tongue" is furious at Finn for having "never [given] me right praise for my deeds" and finds "fault" with his "shape" in so far as "it was not put on the whole of the Fianna the same as on yourself" (Gregory 308). The Fianna express sorrow towards Finn's sudden old age; they believe that he can become young enough with the correct potion, which shows the possibility of rejuvenation. The healer, "Cuilinn of Cuailgne, that some say was Manannan, son of Lir," rescues Finn with "a vessel of red gold" and "no sooner did Finn drink what was in the vessel than his own shape and his appearance came back to him" (Gregory 309). At the location where Finn dropped the vessel, "a tree grew up, and any one that would look at the branches of that tree in the morning, fasting, would have knowledge of all that was to happen on that day" (Gregory 309). This shows the preoccupation with the recovery of youth deep in Irish storytelling. It is thus perhaps not coincidental that Gregory's *The Golden Apple* (1916) is contemporaneous with Yeats's *At the Hawk's Well* (1917), which, although entirely different in dramatic terms from Gregory's play, is also an exploration of rejuvenation (although it does not occur, of course, in Yeats's short play).[34] In this one-act play, an old man who is "all doubled up with age" and a young man named Cuchulain "seek" a well from which "[h]e who drinks, they say, / Of that miraculous water lives for ever" (*VPl*; lines 42, 98, 101–02). However, both the old and young man miss the rising of these healing waters and, as sung by the musicians, "[h]e has lost what may not be found / Till men heap his burial-mound / And all the history ends" (lines 224–26). It shows a preoccupation with ageing and death (and a fantasy of renewal) was part of ancient Irish literature. In their own ways, both Yeats and Gregory drew on this ancient preoccupation. It is significantly interesting that when Yeats and Gregory were writing, this was the element of ancient Irish mythology that they picked up on. Theirs was in some ways a meta-Revivalist practice, reviving ancient stories about revival.

Gregory's Revival drama drew upon the literature of herbal medicine. In Act Two Scene Three of *The Golden Apple*, Simon is again a medium through which Gregory communicates a cure that she had read about. The doctor, whom the giant associates with a metaphorical "coat of healing," is presented as a less reliable medical voice (236; act 1, sc. 4). Simon exclaims, "More enchantments! I having a bit of tow in my ear against the toothache it did not take the same effect upon myself" (260; act 2, sc. 3). It is likely that Gregory discovered this cure from Evelyn's first volume of *Silva* as "[t]here is extracted an oil from the Aſh, by the proceſs on other woods, which is excellent to recover the hearing, ſome drops of it being diſtilled warm into the ears; and for the caries or rot of the bones, toothach, pains in the kidnies and ſpleen, the anointing therewith is moſt ſovereign" (1: 151). In "Herbs, Charms, and Wise Women," a chapter in *Visions and Beliefs in the West of Ireland*, Gregory also mentions a charmed "bit of tow" that is placed "on the person to be cured" (2: 19). Simon suggests cures, grounded in science as well as mythology, that appear to be

[34] Although published in 1917, *At the Hawk's Well* was first performed in London in 1916.

more sensible than the doctor's healing and are likely to earn him more medical respect from the audience as the play progresses.

Gregory's healer was folk stories and Irish and multinational reading material. On 11 October 1912, Gregory wrote in a letter that "[f]or months past I have been suffering terribly from indigestion—only the indigestion is strictly mental" and "[t]o cure it I have 'taken' two big lives of Goethe, one of these in three immense volumes" and she suspects that "[t]he whole cause of my indigestion is an attempt to write two articles which simply won't consent to become finished articles" (*Seventy Years* 497–98). Gregory succeeded in creating a present that would form a new past, blinding others to her controversial history by giving herself and her identity to Ireland and by living for the nation instead of the self. Her pseudo-statement which emanated from this, that she was "one of the happy people without a history," denies her own antecedents and underscores a wounded past; it renounces a bygone time that she hoped would heal up without leaving a visible scar (Gregory, *Seventy Years* 232). This intended historical invisibility, therefore, would perhaps make it easier for her reading public, and indeed Gregory herself, to forget her ancestral ties to colonialism.

* * *

Biddy Early was another important figure in Gregory's self-reinvention. She writes a long chapter in the first series of *Visions and Beliefs in the West of Ireland* (1920) about this role model, "Seers and Healers," which focuses on local practitioners of folk medicine and their healing remedies. In this chapter, Gregory recounts how she visited Early's old house in Feakle in County Clare, which a mother and daughter occupied after Early's death "*twenty years before*" (*Visions and Beliefs* 1: 37). Gregory reports her findings:

> [*The mother*] *told me some of the stories I give below, and showed me the shed where the healer had consulted with her invisible friends. I had already been given by an old patient of hers a 'bottle' prepared for the cure, but which she had been afraid to use. It lies still unopened on a shelf in my storeroom. When I got back at nightfall to the lodge in the woods I found many of the neighbours gathered there, wanting to hear news of 'the Tulla Woman' and to know for certain if she was dead.* (*Visions and Beliefs* 1: 37)

The first subsection within this chapter is fully focussed on Early and her herbal cures, foresight, suggested association with the fairies, and conflict with modern medicine. Gregory's second part of the chapter is named after Mrs. Sheridan in Coole, an elderly woman that "*once met Raftery, the Gaelic poet, at a dance*" and who supplies further knowledge about Early, illness, and fairy-induced sickness (1: 70). At the end of this subdivision, Gregory delineates Mrs. Sheridan's recollection of a supernatural encounter with "a tall man" who is "[f]rom Tir-nan-og" which, he continues, is "not far from you" as "it's near the place where you live," that is, Coole (1: 91). It is interesting that the Land of Youth is here associated with a physical geographic location specific to Gregory and Yeats, which maps their metaphysical ideas to the familiar Coole surroundings.

In the third subsection, Gregory records information about an "*old man*" that she "*called Mr. Saggartan*," who "knew Biddy Early" and whose "uncle was a friend of hers" as well (1: 93, 96–97). Gregory records that his "uncle left [him] the power, and [he] was well able to do them [cures] and did many" (1: 97). Gregory begins this passage with Yeats in mind: "*I was told one day by our doctor, a good fowler and physician, now, alas, passed away, of an old man in Clare who had knowledge of 'the Others,' and I took Mr. Yeats to see him*" (1: 92). The fourth part, "A Great Warrior in the Business," similarly starts with Gregory's concern for Yeats's welfare as "[*i*]*t was on the bounds of Connemara I heard of this healer [Fagan], and went to see his wife in her little rock-built cabin among the boulders, to ask if a cure could be done for Mr. Yeats, who was staying at a friend's house near, and who was at that time troubled by uncertain eyesight*" (1: 103). Gregory describes how both she and Yeats "[*o*]*ne evening later … walked beside the sea to the cottage where* [*they*] *were to meet the healer*" who "*wore a flannel-sleeved waistcoat*" and "*spoke only Irish*" (1: 103). Gregory writes that this healer, called Fagan, "knows in the gathering of the plant what is wrong with the person that is looking for a cure" (1: 110–11). He concluded that one of Yeats's eyes "*was worse than the other*" but that "[i]t's not from *them* [i.e. fairies] the harm came to your eyes" (Gregory 1: 110, 108). R. F. Foster, Yeats's biographer, notes that Gregory "traced folk-remedies for his eyes (dog-violet, boiled in milk: it did not work)" (*Apprentice Mage* 188). This cure was prescribed by the same healer that Gregory introduced to Yeats (who happens to refer to this healer as "Kirwan").

In his chapter "Irish Witch Doctors," situated within the second volume of *Uncollected Prose* (1975), Yeats confirms that Kirwan/Fagan provided him with "a bunch of herbs, which a botanist has since identified as the dog violet, for [him] to drink in boiled milk, which was to be brought to the boil three times"; the healer said that Yeats's optometric ailments were distinct from the fairy "business" (2: 221–22). The final subsection of "Seers and Healers" is based on "Old Deruane" who "*lived in the middle island of Aran, Inishmaan, where I [Gregory] have stayed more than once*" (Gregory 1: 112). Being "*one of the evening visitors to the cottage I [Gregory] stayed in*" whilst she was sojourning there, Old Deruane told her about the "few cures I can do myself" which he got from "two old women" that he met in Manchester, who were "running from Mayo at the time because of the hunger" (Gregory 1: 112, 119). Gregory visited the Aran Isles in an early stage in her personal transformation, and her periodic return to collect folklore evidences her rebirth of the self.

Gregory's self-reinvention—from landlord to arch-Revivalist—has been a matter of interest to scholars. However, intertwined with this change was Gregory's remodelling of herself as a contemporary Biddy Early. Letters quoted earlier in this chapter reveal her dispensing of cough cures. In a letter to Blunt, the poet who visited Egypt with her in December 1881, Gregory writes that the poor people "believe[d] that I can cure them of all diseases" (*Seventy Years* 232). This language that she uses to portray her neighbour's perceptions of her is strikingly similar to the words describing Early in the first series of *Visions and Beliefs*. In this work, Gregory records that Early knows "a cure for all sicknesses" (1: 51). Even though Gregory records statements that paint Early as a mercenary character, this does not mean that she necessarily believed them. Rather, Gregory saw in Early a native healer of Ireland. It is recorded that Early, according to informant Dolly Steward, "could cure [whooping cough] with thyme tea" (qtd. in Ryan 33). From 1880, Gregory inhabited the same place and space as Early, just six years after Early's death in 1874. The vicinity's healing plants were on Gregory's doorstep, but Early had to travel from Clare to Coole for some of her ingredients.

In "Seers and Healers," Gregory records an informant's account that guarantees her knowledge of Early's associations with cures local to Coole. The Spinning-Woman reveals to Gregory that this famous folk healer "slept in Ballylee mill last night, and that there was a cure for all things in the world between the two wheels there" (1: 52). Due to the elderly Mr. Saggarton's information, Gregory later confirms that this refers to the healing moss that only cures fairy-induced illnesses (1: 99). Meda Ryan states that "[m]oss had many curative properties and Biddy was openly seen picking bits of this tufty growth from around the wheel of the mill-stream of Ballylee, beside the [t]ower where W. B. Yeats came to live later" (33). Through Gregory, Early's legacy strode forward into the modern world of medicine; even though Gregory did not claim to possess magical abilities, she continued Early's practice of herbalism.

* * *

There is a strong possibility that Gregory's cough cure was the forester's panacea, a universal remedy that she was very likely to have come across in her reading and the materials for which she certainly held in her environs. In her library at Coole, Gregory owned gardener John Evelyn's (1620–1706) *Silva; or, A Discourse of Forest-Trees* (1786), a two-volume edition that she handpicked as one of her favourite books. William Gregory wrote in his will that Augusta could keep six books that belonged in his library in Coole, although he later left her all of them.[35] Gregory contemplated the hypothetical situation of "[h]ad I inherited that choice of six" and decided that "Evelyn's *Silva* also, with its beautiful coloured plates of larch and 'Silver Firr'" would have found a home in this quota (*Coole* 20).[36] Based on this evidence that Gregory valued *Silva*, Anna Pilz deduces that "[c]onsidering that Gregory held this book in such high regard, we can surmise that it was likely a constant companion, frequently consulted and re-read" ("Lady Gregory's 'Tree Planting'" 88). There is a strong possibility that Gregory was deeply familiar with this book's contents. In the second volume, there is a cough cure that corresponds with both Gregory's reading and the herbal ingredients available to her: the forester's panacea. Evelyn declares this to be a remedy that "I have often made for my poor neighbours" (*Silva* 2: 13). Similarly, Gregory prepared cough cures for her less fortunate neighbours in Coole, an idea that stemmed from both her heterogeneous reading and medicinal environment.

Most likely, she used Evelyn's instructions in *Silva* to correctly mix the forester's panacea. The main ingredient of this cure for coughs, amongst other illnesses, is the healing berries from the juniper tree:

[35] Evelyn's *Silva* is listed in *Catalogue of Printed Books Formerly in the Library at Coole: The Property of the Lady Gregory Estate*, an inventory of the family's books that auctioneers sold in 1972 (23; Sotheby).

[36] Gregory pondered, "But if, as seems likely, I am now, through changes, to be divorced from these companionable shelves, I sometimes ponder which among the volumes should I choose from their long accustomed places to go with me for the scanty years or days of eyesight and understanding that may remain" (*Coole* 17).

> The berries afford (befides a tolerable pepper) one of the moft univerfal remedies in the world to our crazy Forefter. Being fwallowed only, they inftantly appeafe the wind-cholic; and, in decoction, they are moft fovereign againft an inveterate cough. The water is a moft fingular fpecific againft the gravel in the reins [i.e. kidneys]; but all is comprehended in the virtue of the theriacle, or electuary, which I have often made for my poor neighbours, and may well be termed the forefter's panacea againft the ftone, rheum, phthific, dropfy, jaundice, inward impofthumes, nay, palfy, gout, and the plague itfelf. (Evelyn, *Silva* 2: 13–14)

The berries are thus heated in water or beer, and an electuary is created with the addition of a sweetener, such as honey or sugar. Around the turloughs at Coole, which are "seasonal lakes," the *juniperus communis* is one of the "heath communities" that "have developed over the limestone pavement" ("Nature & Wildlife").[37] Hence its Latinate name and according to Volume One Part Two of Philip Miller's *The Gardener's and Botanist's Dictionary* (1807), another work that belonged in Gregory's library, this juniper is "common in all the northern parts of Europe" and different species grow elsewhere (Miller, "Juniperus" sec. 7; *Catalogue* 42). Not only is the remedy universal and therefore widely accessible, Evelyn also distributed this exact cure to his own neighbours, a practice that parallels Gregory's in her own district.

The juniper had magical connotations and Gregory came across this plant in Inchy, a County Clare town. She visited the fellow writer and botanist Emily Lawless on 26 November 1926, and she recalls that "[w]e sat among the juniper bushes and rocks one afternoon at Inchy when she [Lawless] was staying here" (*Lady Gregory's Journals* 219). In *Visions and Beliefs*, Gregory records a story, told by a man called John Mangan, about "a bush the form of an umbrella" that was "growing close by the water" at "Inchy Weir" (2: 229). The same story features in the "Woods, Visions, and the Lake" chapter in *Coole* (1971), a printed collection of some of Gregory's manuscripts, in which Gregory writes, "It was over at Inchy weir also, beyond that field of rocks covered by spreading juniper, that as a man still living told me, he and his brother had gone one day in their boyhood to catch a horse" (95). This confirms that the "bush the form of an umbrella" that she refers to in her folklore collectanea and manuscripts is most likely to be a juniper. Yeats reports the same story in *A Celtic*

[37] For a list of trees and plants that grow around the Coole waters, in the woods, and in Gregory's garden, see the *Coole Park Nature Reserve* website: www.coolepark.ie.

Twilight (1902) in so far as "[a] man told me that one day, when he was a boy, he and another boy went to catch a horse in a certain field, full of boulders and bushes of hazel and creeping juniper and rock-roses, that is where the lake-side is for a little clear of the woods" (*Mythologies* 41).[38] Aside from Gregory describing the juniper as "spreading" and Yeats depicting it as "creeping" across the landscapes, the two versions are strikingly similar. In this folk narrative, the siblings venture to find a horse but instead discover a bush; they bet that if they "fling a pebble on to that bush it will stay on it" due to its "matted" appearance (Yeats 41). However, as soon as the stone "hit the bush there came out of it the most beautiful music that ever was heard" (Yeats 41). In Yeats's account, this fairy bush could be "hazel" or the "creeping juniper" or the "rock-roses" (41). As Gregory's version only mentions the juniper, it is possible that the magical bush is a *juniperus communis* and is therefore planted in mythology as well as traditional medicine; it is an ingredient for the Irish Literary Revival as well as a legitimate universal healing for multitudinous illnesses.

In folklore, both in Ireland and around the world, the juniper had mythological and medical associations. Richard Folkard, a nineteenth-century horticulturalist, states that the juniper is a "protective tree" that repels illness and evil (395). He also states, "The old herbalists recommended the berries of the [j]uniper for use as counter poisons" (Folkard 397). Patrick Logan notes that the "juice of juniper berries" was "used simply as a diueretic" (*Making the Cure* 38–39). Muiris Ó hUiginn, an informant for *The Schools' Manuscript Collection* (*NFCS*), notes a juniper remedy used in County Donegal: "Aiteannach a' Chnuic (Juniper). Maith ag casachtas. É a bhruith agus an súgh a ól. Treacal agus siúcra buidhe a chur fríd an t-sugh" ("Luibheanna" 60).[39] In English, this translates as "Juniper. Good for coughing. Boil it and drink the juice. Add treacle and yellow sugar through the juice" ("Luibheanna" 60; my translation). Although Ó hUiginn does not label it as such, this is clearly the same

[38] It is possible that Gregory gave Yeats this story so that he could make money from its publication when he was in financial difficulty. Kohfeldt informs that Yeats "wrote up the stories from the notes she [Gregory] gave him and they were published by the editors to whom Augusta introduced him" (105). Therefore, instead of donating her juniper medicine in this case, she supplied Yeats with the mythical and literary properties of the plant.

[39] *NFCS* 1059: 60; Muiris Ó hUiginn (72), Ardara, County Donegal. Collector: Pádraic Ó Breisleáin, An Mhín Mhór (school), Meenmore, County Donegal, 1932. Teacher: Pádraic Ó Breisleáin.

substance as the forester's panacea. Both Coole library and folk medicine provided similar cures.

* * *

Gregory completed her ten-year transformation as a new woman with a fresh vision for her life. She fostered a deliberate selective memory and self-selective process, which enabled her to forget her past and become a spiritual self-portrait of Cathleen Ni Houlihan and a medical mirror image of Biddy Early. Based on the rejuvenated *cailleach* and the folk healer, Gregory put into practice a new lifestyle that focussed on reviving Ireland, restoring the health of her neighbourhood, and challenging colonialism. Ó Crualaoich's identification of the *cailleach* as a healer that can offer different well-being services provides a new angle with which to view this traditional Irish character. Gregory, too, had a multi-faceted identity. As a *bean ghlúine* or midwife, she brought a revived Ireland into the world; as a *bean feasa* or wise woman, she mixed medicines for her neighbours. Her own rejuvenation and Ireland's were inextricably linked.

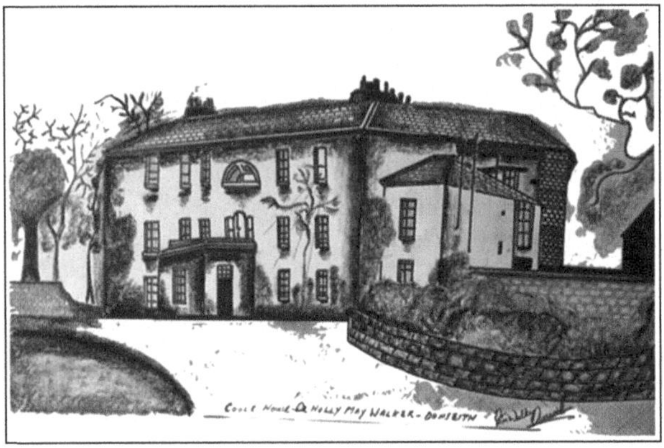

Coole House

CHAPTER 5

The Language of Healing Herbs

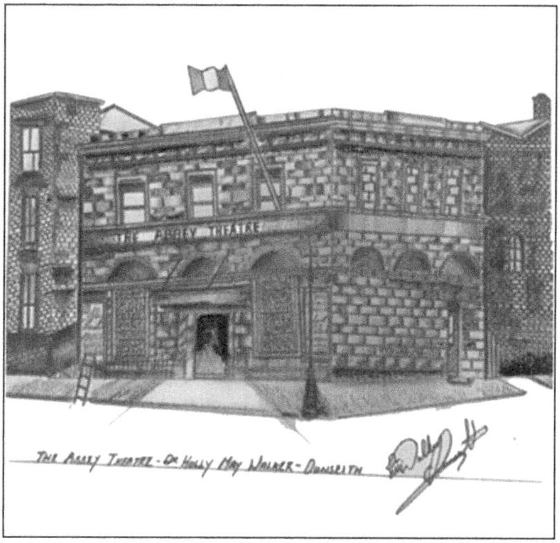

The Abbey Theatre

H. M. Walker-Dunseith, *Traditional Medicine in the Irish Literary Revival*, New Directions in Irish and Irish American Literature,
https://doi.org/10.1007/978-3-031-82459-3_5

In William Butler Yeats and Lady Augusta Gregory's collaborative play *The Pot of Broth* (1904), ostensibly a light farce, a beggar visits a couple and convinces them that a stone he carries is magical and can be boiled to make broth. As he demonstrates this "magic," there is a crucial passage in which the tramp asks for herbs. By reading this passage alongside Gregory's other writings on herbs, and in the light of her association with the healer Bridget Ruane, we can understand the tramp's role in the play better, and the role of non-elite women like Ruane in the creation of the culture of the Revival. Gregory's "Herb-Healing" chapter in *Poets and Dreamers: Studies and Translations from the Irish* (1902) and the "Herbs, Charms, and Wise Women" section in the second series of *Visions and Beliefs in the West of Ireland* (1920)[1] throw light on *The Pot of Broth.* Many of the herbs that Gregory lists and describes in these folklore collections are repurposed as literary ingredients that she and Yeats mix into *The Pot of Broth*, as well as other plays, where they create a symbolic language of healing herbs.

There is a metanarrative running through Yeats's and Gregory's works and drama: they aim to cure and heal the world from damaging, shallow materialism and introduce a new era in which the heart is valued over the head. This is the mindset that led to them founding a national theatre in Dublin at the start of a new century. Though this is often thought about in primarily political terms, they also had a view to creating a new world. Both writers wanted a global salvation, an act of remaking and rejuvenating the world-mind. This project of rejuvenation and recovery tied in with nationalistic beliefs, but also extended into the wider world too. As such, the healing herbs the beggar asks for in *The Pot of Broth* are more than just incidental. They are an element in a project to heal Ireland from its afflictions of materialism and greed.

The artist-healer is central to Gregory, as ascertained by James Pethica. In his introduction to *Collaborative One-Act Plays, 1901–1903: Cathleen Ni Houlihan, The Pot of Broth, The Country of the Young, Heads or Harps:*

[1] The second edition of *Poets and Dreamers: Studies and Translations from the Irish* (1903) and both series of *Visions and Beliefs in the West of Ireland* (1920) are physical texts that are held in the National Library of Ireland (NLI) in Dublin. Located in the W. B. Yeats Library collection, the NLI website describes *Poets and Dreamers* as having "[m]anuscript notes on sheet pasted on the title page, also on pages 77, 153 and endpapers" ("Poets and Dreamers"). In terms of "[p]hysical description," this book has "4 preliminary leaves, 254 pages; 21 cm" ("Poets and Dreamers"). Both the first series and the second series of *Visions and Beliefs* have a "[f]rontispiece" that is "a photograph of a picture by Robert Gregory" and the NLI website frames the "[p]hysical description" as "2 volumes: illustrations; frontispieces; 20 cm" ("Visions and Beliefs").

Manuscript Materials (2006), a collection of manuscripts that tracks the changes in the collaborative plays, Pethica argues that "[a] core vision of the artist as a healer who comes to repair the social economy or to inspire others, but who then typically withdraws unobtrusively, would underpin her principal work as a dramatist, and also inform her optimistic core conception of the theater movement as a venue in which artists such as Yeats, herself, and others might model beneficial social and political change for Ireland" (lvi). Pethica mentions three plays in which Gregory casts a healer as the protagonist: the poet Raftery in *The Marriage* (1902); the ragged man in *The Rising of the Moon* (1903); and Jesus Christ, who is the Divine Physician and the Greatest Healer, in *The Travelling Man* (1905) (lvi).[2] In the Yeats-Gregory collaborative play *The Pot of Broth*, however, the protagonist tramp is presented as far from a healer figure although he pretends to have a substantial knowledge of herbal medicine. Pethica notices, "The Tramp's allusions to the beneficial properties of herbs . . . closely parallel material in Lady Gregory's essay 'Herb-Healing,' originally published in *The Westminster Budget* in 1900, and reprinted in her 1903 volume *Poets and Dreamers*" (xlvi). I argue that Gregory's reference to herbs becomes a language that is not only used as a form of communication in this collaborative play, but it also re-surfaces in her other independent plays.

The Pot of Broth is a Yeats-Gregory collaboration that showcases Gregory's knowledge that she learned from Bridget Ruane who was a local Irish herbalist and a key source for Gregory's "Herb-Healing" chapter. This one-act play, on its surface, explores for comic effect themes of poverty, parsimoniousness, and credulity. A tramp arrives at John and Sibby Coneely's cottage in search for food and tells them that a magical stone is a renewable food source that can make "a good drop of broth or a bit of stirabout, or a drop of poteen itself" (lines 194–96; act 1). The tramp places the stone in "a pot with a drop of boiling water in it" and advises that it is effective to add "a bit of an herb for fear the enchantment might slip away from it" (lines 149–50, 157–58). To this end, he asks the couple if they have three herbs that were thought to be magic herbs with miraculous powers: the slanlus, fearavan, and the athair-talav. The couple do not have access to the slanlus and fearavan, but the athair-talav grows in their garden. Nevertheless, the tramp settles for "*a couple of good*

[2] *The Marriage* (1902) is the product of a collaboration between Gregory and Douglas Hyde. This work can be found in Gregory's *Poets and Dreamers* (1903) in which she identifies it as one of An Craoibh's, meaning Douglas Hyde's, plays (216–35). Gregory's independent works, *The Rising of the Moon* (1903) and *The Travelling Man* (1905), are printed in editor Mary FitzGerald's *Selected Plays by Lady Gregory* (1983).

handfuls of the cabbage and onions and puts them in" to the pot alongside other ingredients for the broth (line 171). When Sibby asks the tramp if he would give them the stone, he replies that he would only exchange the stone with a pot as "I never can keep a pot with me" (lines 308–09). In compliance, Sibby responds with two imperative commands: "Give me the loan of the stone itself, and I'll engage I'll keep a pot for it" and "[w]ait now till I'll make some offer to you" (lines 319–21). The tramp, however, decides that "I'll ask nothing at all for it" yet ironically "*takes up the chicken*" and "[*t*]*akes the* [*b*]*ottle*" of whiskey before he leaves their cottage (lines 333, 337, 339). At the resolution, Sibby exclaims that "I'll be as rich as Biddy Early before I die!" and John recommends to her that "[m]aybe you'd best put the stone in the pot again" (lines 345–46, 352–53). The dramatic irony occurs in the audience's awareness that the stone is a prop for deception rather than a magical cure for hunger.

Following an elaborate and dramatic listing of various herbs from "Herb-Healing," the tramp settles for the simple "leaves beside me" that "will do well enough" and "[*h*]*e takes a couple of good handfuls of the cabbage and onions and puts them in*" the pot (line 171). Though a simple enough playlet, it partakes of the metanarrative that is visible in so many of Yeats's and Gregory's theatrical works at the turn of the twentieth century. Through their own greed and materialism, John and Sibby Coneely are confounded. Their dull and shallow materialism is defeated by the attractive intellectual power of the tramp. Ireland was a wellspring for this transformative vision, but it was not its limit. The settings Yeats and Gregory employed were Irish; the language their protagonists spoke was distinctive to Ireland, yet the kind of recovery that Yeats and Gregory envisioned would have relevance far beyond the country's shores.

* * *

Bridget Ruane was a healer, local to Gregory, whose knowledge was inherited from her brother. In "Herb-Healing," an inventory of cures that Gregory learnt from Ruane herself, Gregory describes her as "a respectable-looking old woman, dressed in the red petticoat and blue cloak of the country-people" (111). Although her birth date seems to be unknown, Gregory certifies that "she died last winter" in her chapter "Herb-Healing," which she wrote in 1900 and then published in *Poets and Dreamers* in 1902 (120). Ruane was therefore likely to have died in winter 1899, not long after she wrote a letter to Gregory on 28 September 1899 about "one of the Fathers, a Saint" in London who could "tell me his remedies" (111). This letter, written at the very end of Ruane's life, would feature as the frontispiece for Gregory's chapter that listed this healer's cures and therefore kept her memory alive. Ruane mentions in the letter that a patient was sent "back to Gort, here to me," a location in walking distance from Coole Park, which suggests that this is where she lived and mixed remedies and dispensed cures to people who came to her for help (111). Ruane was an accessible muse who gave Gregory the materials from which to craft a new language and set of preoccupations, and the tools with which to reshape herself as an inheritor and communicator of herbal knowledge.

Gregory's chapter about this healer appears to be the most substantial source of information on Ruane in existence. In *Visions and Beliefs*, Gregory alludes to this earlier section: "*I have told in 'Poets and Dreamers' of old Bridget Ruane who came and gave me my first knowledge of the healing power of certain plants, some it seemed having a natural and some a mysterious power*" (2: 3). Although Ruane is not mentioned in the *Dictionary of Irish Biography* (2021) and is less famous than Biddy Early, she was something of a local legend amongst the people in counties Clare and Galway, and the surrounding areas.[3] Before Gregory published her writing, Ruane's legend lived on through word of mouth in the oral Irish tradition. In "Mickey Filler and the Tansey Wreath," a narrative about Ruane's grandson that is placed in a collection of folk tales titled *Ghosts in Irish Houses* (1947), James Reynolds avers that "[i]n all the countryside, even into the counties of Cork, Tipperary, and Kerry, the name of Bridget Ruane was a household word" and that "[t]he miracles of healing performed by Bridget were well known by all the poor and hapless" (41). Reynolds reveals that "[t]he children roundabout did not call Mickey's grandmother by her right name; they called her Biddy Early" (41). This was echoed many years before in 1900 in *Poets and Dreamers*, where Gregory records a conversation with "[a] neighbour whom I asked about Bridget Ruane and her brother," who revealed that "[s]ome people call her 'Biddy Early' (after a famous witch-doctor)" (114). Ruane's service to

[3] Although Bridget Ruane's name was well known in the west of Ireland, there are a severe dearth of accounts about her, and she remains a highly under-researched member of Irish society. Other places that I have searched and could not find her include *The Main Manuscript Collection* (*NFC*) and *The Schools' Manuscript Collection* (*NFCS*). In *The Schools' Manuscript Collection*, there are three accounts that feature the name Bridget Ruane, but they are not likely to be referring to the healer.

Gregory was to teach her traditional medicine; Gregory preserved her medical memory in written format, without which, Ruane would most likely be lost in the shadow of Early.

In Gregory's "Herb-Healing," a chapter in her collection of folklore essays and translations *Poets and Dreamers*, Ruane is a tutelary spirit. The chapter opens with a letter from Ruane, addressed to the "Honourable Lady Gregory," and dated on 28 September 1899 (111). In this letter, Ruane mythologises the origins of her knowledge as follows:

> I, Bridget Ruane, wish to inform you that there is in the Oratory in London one of the Fathers, a Saint. I do not know his name; but there was a young woman of the name of Meara; she got two falls and could get no cure. She went to London and found this holy man; and he sent her back to Gort, here to me, and I cured her. If your honourable Ladyship could make him out, it would be a wonderful thing, and a great happiness to many a weary heart, and the great God would have it in store for you and your son. May you enjoy many happy days together is the prayer of your humble servant, [Bridget Ruane]. (Gregory 111)

When Gregory "went down to see the writer" in person, Ruane again asked Gregory the same question and explained that she could not perform all cures, but claimed the ability to resurrect people from death using the slanlus herb:

> Now if you could find out the name of that Saint through the press, he'd tell me his remedies; and between us, all the world would be cured. For I can't do all cures, though there are a great many I can do. I cured Michael Miscail when the doctor couldn't do it, and a woman in Gort that was paralyzed, and her two sons that were stretched. For I can bring back the dead with some of the herbs our Lord was brought back with, the *Garalus* and the *Slanlus*. But there are some things I can't do. I can't help anyone that has got a stroke from the Queen or the Fool of the Forth. (111–12)

Yeats glosses the mysterious final phrase in his essay "The Queen and the Fool," in which he states that he has "heard one Hearne, a witch-doctor, who is on the border of Clare and Galway, say that … 'every household' of Faery" has one of each of these classes of fairy, and that these entities have unusual power (*Mythologies* 75). It is unknown as to whether Gregory attempted to fulfil Ruane's request, but it is certain that Ruane's herbal knowledge was a source of intrigue for her. In fact, Gregory remarks that

"I asked her to teach me some of her fragments of Druids' wisdom, the healing power of herbs" (112). At the dawn of the twentieth century, Gregory was trying to recover a pre-Christian past. Ruane, according to Gregory, "came another day, and brought some herbs, and sorted them out on a table" and told Gregory about each one (112).

Gregory became a student and apprentice when Ruane taught her about the medical properties of herbs and passed down her knowledge. Her story began with a fairy-tale-like origin of her family's special knowledge that reveals a metaphorical truth but not a literal or written truth. It is a metaphor for those who would deprecate traditional healers:

> It was my brother got the knowledge of cures from a book that was thrown down before him on the road. What language was it written in? What language would it be but Irish? May be it was God gave it to him, and may be it was the *other people*. He was a fine strong man; and he weighed fifteen stone; and he went to England, and there he cured all the world, so that the doctors had no way of living. So one time he got in a ship to go to America; and the doctors had bad men engaged to shipwreck him out of the ship; he wasn't drowned, but he was broken to pieces on the rocks, and the book was lost along with him. (112)

Nevertheless, Gregory notes Ruane's claims that her brother "taught me a good deal out of it" and that "[s]o I know all herbs, and I do a good many cures; and I have brought a good many children home to the world, and never lost one, or one of the women that bore them" (112). In a list format, Gregory wrote down every cure and definition that Ruane had discussed, thus creating a chapter of medical lexicon. Many of the herbs that Gregory mentions in her plays come from the short chapter, "Herb-Healing," which is dated 1900. At the same time as she was learning of herbs from Ruane, these healing plants sprouted in her literary work.

* * *

Gregory's knowledge that she learnt from Ruane's herbal expertise is traceable in *The Pot of Broth*. The pivotal moment in the play's action happens when the tramp lists three herbs that could be added into the pot with the stone. The audience will have seen the tramp ask for the slanlus, fearavan, and athair-talav. They would have even witnessed his provision of specific details about how to gather the first two herbs that he requested from the couple, and then watched him choose vegetables instead. This scene demonstrates Gregory's knowledge of traditional medicine, which flavoured the joint-authored play and provided Yeats with knowledge that was unique to his collaborator.

Addressing the miserly Sibby, a resident of the cottage, the tramp raises the issue of herbs: "You wouldn't have a bit of Slanlus in the house, ma'am, that was cut with a black-handled knife?" (lines 159–61). In "Herb-Healing," Gregory similarly capitalises "*Slanlus*," groups it as one of "the best of the herbs," and writes Ruane's definition in a seemingly word-for-word fashion: "Here are the *Slanlus* (plantain) and the *Garblus* (dandelion); and these would cure the wide world; and it was these brought our Lord from the Cross, … His Mother and Mary and Joseph gathered these herbs and cured His wounds" (114). Slanlus is therefore associated with revival and resurrection, a key theme in Gregory and Yeats's shared plays.

It is very likely that Gregory is responsible for this herbal section in the play. Yeats's poor health at this time meant that a large amount of the work in writing this play fell to her. James Pethica notes that "[m]uch of the work was evidently completed by dictation... with Lady Gregory occupying a secretarial role" due to Yeats's poor eyesight (*Collaborative One-Act Plays* xlv-xlvi). In a letter to Blunt, dated on 13 September 1902, Gregory writes that her collaborator's "eyes are bad this year, & he has to dictate almost everything to me, plays & letters" (qtd. in Pethica, *Collaborative One-Act Plays* xlvi). However, this did not mean that Gregory was merely Yeats's scribe. Pethica also states, "As in *Cathleen ni Houlihan*, Lady Gregory's influence on *The Pot of Broth* registers in the distinctive 'Kiltartan' speech the characters use, in the use of folklore materials drawn from her gatherings, and also in narrative structure" and writes in the footnotes that "[t]he Tramp's allusions to the beneficial properties of herbs … closely parallel material in Lady Gregory's essay 'Herb-Healing,' originally published in *The Westminster Budget* in 1900, and reprinted in her 1903 volume *Poets and Dreamers*" (xlvi). Gregory is therefore putting her herbal knowledge to comedic use.

It appears that Gregory almost felt she had to put herself in second place as a comedy writer in deference to Yeats's serious tone. This has been argued by Garry Hynes in an interview for the *Irish Women's Writing (1880–1920) Network* titled *In Conversation with Garry Hynes* (2021). The interviewer Anna Pilz asks Hynes about the Druid Theatre's

DruidGregory project.[4] She states that Gregory has "always been seen as filling in at the Abbey, providing comedy to offset the more verse-heavy work by especially Yeats" (00:37:59–00.38.11; my transcription). She also quotes Gregory's lecture, "On Making a Play": "the circumstances of our theatre have forced me to write comedy; the strain of the attention necessary for listening to verse requires a relaxing afterwards" (00:38:12–27; my transcription). Pilz comments that "it's the sense of lean-back; it's an undemanding part of the programme but, in DruidGregory, obviously she becomes the main act; she's no longer a filler at all" (00.38.29–33; my transcription). Pilz asks Hynes a question: "What, in your sense, by producing the plays together, what kind of key themes become apparent that speak to the twenty-first century audience?" (00:38:40–49; my transcription). In response to this question, Hynes says that "I think her own presence looms large in her work and obviously the ideas of the time and the nationalism of the time are very much there" (00:38:53–00:39:05; my transcription). Hynes also notes Gregory's "utter delight in Irish legend" and "her delight in covering something that wasn't available without somebody like her listening to and getting the stories from the people around her … I think she's dazzled by that and she's dazzled by these legends and stories and she's so thrilled to be able to use them as a subject for plays" (00:39:08–47; my transcription). Yeats was viewed as the serious artist, and so Gregory puts herself in second place as a comedy writer. She pursued folklore-learning and made it an element of comedy even though, arguably, comedy was not her first love. Reading Gregory's prose work alongside *The Pot of Broth* shows how Gregory put very serious learning to comic ends.

By the time she came to co-write *The Pot of Broth*, Lady Gregory had already written a sincere work of herbalism that was embedded in *Poets and Dreamers* in 1903, and she was yet to expand her findings in *Visions and Beliefs* in 1920. It is the same material in *The Pot of Broth* as in her herbalist collections but, in the collaborative writing of the play, the herbs are treated in a light-hearted manner:

> SIBBY. And is that all you have to put in it?
>
> TRAMP. Nothing at all but that, — only maybe a bit of an herb for fear the enchantment might slip away from it. You wouldn't have a bit of the Slán-lus in the house ma'am, that was cut with a black-handled knife?

[4] DruidGregory, DruidSynge, and DruidMurphy are respective projects whereby a selection of each author's plays are performed by the *Druid Theatre Company*.

SIBBY. No indeed, I have none of that in the house.

TRAMP. Or a bit of the Fearaván that was picked when the wind was from the north?

SIBBY. No, indeed, I'm sorry there's none.

TRAMP. Or a sprig of the Athair-talav, the father of herbs?

JOHN. There's plenty of it by the hedge. I'll go out and get it for you.

TRAMP. O, don't mind taking so much trouble; those leaves beside me will do well enough. (*Collaborative One-Act Plays* lines 191–212)

Following this, a stage direction reads that "[*h*]*e takes a couple of good handfuls of the cabbage and onions and puts them in*" the pot (line 212). In the end, these herbs do not form part of the pot of broth, and instead vegetables are used in their place.[5] Even when the "sprig of the Athair-talav" is near at hand, Gregory's voice speaks through the tramp as he instructs John not to "mind taking so much trouble" (lines 206, 210–11). The tramp is pretending to have knowledge of herbs and healing, and he is boiling up the stone and feigning that it is going to be food. The comedy emanates from two elements that occur simultaneously: language and actions. It is a sum of the division between what the audience are being told versus what they are seeing on the stage. Gregory is using the significant gap between herbal knowledge and comedy. In her collaborations with Yeats, however, she thought that she had to be the comedian, and this changes her relationship to her material. Therefore, Gregory was most likely desiring to write a play of her own at this point in her career, hence the profuse herbal content in her later play *The Golden Apple* (1916).

In the interview *In Conversation with Garry Hynes*, Hynes states that Gregory is "vastly underrated," which prompts a question from Pilz: "What do you think has shaped that underratedness or that occlusion from the canon shall we say?" (00:13:44–58; my transcription). In response, Hynes says that "I think there were a lot of reasons" and "I don't think she helped herself in the sense that she allowed Yeats to take credit for things" (00:14:00–07; my transcription). She avers that "living in Yeats's shadow when Yeats was alive must have been difficult" and she

[5] The punctuation changes in the different sources are displayed in the footnotes on pages 107–08 of "1904 Published Text with Collations, 1902–1904" in Pethica's *Collaborative One-Act Plays* (2006).

emphasises "the fact that she was a woman" who was "doing what would be seen as male things like founding and running a theatre" (00:14:08–33; my transcription). She adds that Gregory "had so many fights with Yeats about finance and she fights with the Abbey board" and that "this was a woman who, every evening, was checking the size of the house and thrilled when she was forced to put out extra seats into the stalls, and this was her daily life" (00:14:34–55; my transcription). Hynes points out that these everyday tasks that Gregory performed are not widely known (00:14:56–00:15:02). Gregory perhaps thought that she had to be the comedian due to patriarchy and her role as a woman at the time, which is a plausible reason for her taking second place.

Gregory treats the spelling of the herbs with the utmost care and attention. Firstly, she spells slanlus as "Slan-lus" in the original typescript version from before October 1902 (Yeats and Gregory, *Collaborative One-Act Plays* 107). This variant spelling also occurs in the play's first official publication in *The Hour-Glass and Other Plays: Being Volume Two of Plays for an Irish Theatre* in January 1904 (Yeats 97).[6] Gregory would later change the spelling to "Slán-lus" in March 1904, when the play was revised and republished in *The Hour-Glass, Cathleen ni Houlihan, The Pot of Broth: Being Volume Two of Plays for an Irish Theatre* (Yeats 71).[7] Secondly, Gregory spells fearavan as "Faravan" in the transcript and first publication; this becomes "Fearaván" in the March 1904 edition (Yeats, *Hour-Glass and Other Plays* 98; Yeats, *Hour-Glass* 71). Thirdly, Pethica notes that the athair-talav herb was originally spelt as "Ahartalav" in the typescript and it was then changed to "Áhartalav" using ink in the same source (*Collaborative One-Act Plays* 108). Gregory would change this back to "Ahartalav" in the January 1904 publication of *The Hour-Glass and Other Plays* (Yeats 98). She then decided upon "Athair-talav" in the 1905 republication of *The Hour-Glass, Cathleen ni Houlihan, The Pot of Broth* (Yeats 72).[8] In *Poets and Dreamers*, the herbs are italicised as "*Slanlus*," "*Fearaban*," and "*Athair-talav*" (Gregory 112; 113). In *Visions and Beliefs*, they are presented as "*slanlus*," "*fearaban*," and "*atair-talam*" (Gregory 2: 5; 7).

[6] See Yeats and Gregory's *Collaborative One-Act Plays* (2006), edited by Pethica (107). Also, see Yeats's *The Hour-Glass and Other Plays: Being Volume Two of Plays for an Irish Theatre* (1904), specifically page 97.

[7] See Yeats's *The Hour-Glass, Cathleen ni Houlihan, The Pot of Broth* (1904; A. H. Bullen).

[8] Peruse Yeats's *The Hour-Glass, Cathleen ni Houlihan, The Pot of Broth* (1905; Maunsel).

Gregory's attention to detail, even to the minute level of spelling, reveals her meticulous attitude towards these herbs.

Gregory's punctilious treatment of the noun phrase "an herb" is also of interest as this shows that her conscientiousness for herbalism extended to even the smallest building blocks of grammar. In response to Sibby's question about whether the tramp only had to place the stone in the pot, the tramp replies, "Nothing at all but that, — only maybe a bit of an herb for fear the enchantment might slip away from it" (*Collaborative One-Act Plays* lines 193–95). Gregory wrote "a herb" in the early typescript (*Collaborative One-Act Plays* 107). However, she omitted articles altogether in *The Hour-Glass and Other Plays* when she simply wrote "a bit of herb" (97). By March 1904, Gregory had changed this to "a bit of an herb" in *The Hour-Glass, Cathleen ni Houlihan, The Pot of Broth* (71). This decision to use "an" was queried in "[a] set of page proofs for *The Collected Plays of W. B. Yeats*, 1934" (Pethica, *Collaborative One-Act Plays* xvii; Wade, *Bibliography* 180–01).[9] Either Thomas Mark, who was the reader and editor for Macmillan and Company in 1934, or an unknown member of the publishing team or Yeats himself questioned Gregory's choice of indefinite article to accompany her treasured "herb." Pethica notes that "an" was "*circled and queried but query then del*" (*Collaborative One-Act Plays* 107). This means that this unique phrasing stood out to the editing eye, but it was then retracted in favour of Gregory's choice of syntax and grammar.

Gregory perhaps justified her phrasing of "an herb" using local Irish usage. It is likely that some form of communication occurred at some point between the query and subsequent deletion, which probably involved Gregory, Yeats, and the editors. In both "Herb-Healing" and "Herbs, Charms, and Wise Women," Gregory wrote down accounts that were spoken to her by the local people, many of which are recorded as saying "an herb." For example, in "Herb-Healing," Gregory writes about "[a]nother neighbour, who has herself some reputation as an herb-doctor" and an "old man," later identified as "*Old Heffernan*" in "Herbs, Charms, and Wise Women," who claimed that "[t]he best herb-doctor I ever knew was Connolly up at Kilbecanty" and said, "I had a lump on the thigh one

[9] Pethica notes, "The proofs are marked 'First proof' and date-stamped with various dates between July 5, 1934, and August 9, 1934, and marked up with corrections in the hands of Yeats, Thomas Mark, and possibly others, including revisions to *Cathleen ni Houlihan* and *The Pot of Broth*" (*Collaborative One-Act Plays* xvii).

time, and my father went to him, and he gave him *an herb* for it; but he told him not to come into the house by the door the wind would be blowing in at" (*Poets and Dreamers* 115–16; emphasis added; *Visions and Beliefs* 2: 11). In "Herbs, Charms, and Wise Women," Gregory wrote down an account by Mrs. Cloonan, an informant who gathered herbs to be used as medicine (2: 10–11). She was careful not to meddle with herbs that were believed to contain a "*pishogue*" (which is "[a] spell, incantation, or charm") and therefore "harm" (*Visions and Beliefs* 2: 11; "Pishogue"; *OED*). Mrs. Cloonan, as recorded by Gregory, said, "I used to be gathering *an herb* one time for the Bishop that lived at Loughmore, dandelion it was" and "[t]here are two sorts, the white that has no harm in it, that's what I used to be gathering, and the red that has a *pishogue* in it, but I left that alone" (*Visions and Beliefs* 2: 11; first emphasis added). Another informant named James Mangan tells Gregory that "[f]or a swelling in the throat it's *an herb* would be used" (2: 19; emphasis added). It is evident that Gregory heard "an herb" from the people around her and she took the opportunity to take this phrase from her surroundings and channel it, not only into her folklore collections, but also into her playwriting.

Gregory's deliberate choice to write "an herb" is perhaps a feature of her Kiltartan dialect, which has thus far been overlooked by scholars. She most likely heard this noun phrase from her folklore-collecting travels, and it appears that she wrote down exactly what she heard. Gregory does not conform to standard English grammar, which prescribes that the indefinite article "an" is placed prior to the sound of a vowel. This suggests that the "h" is dropped in "an herb," which means that Gregory is supporting an Irish rather than English pronunciation. The Kiltartan dialect, which Gregory derived from the Irish spoken in a nearby townland, already features prominently in the play. Whilst "a herb" is still used in *Poets and Dreamers* and *Visions and Beliefs*, alongside its Kiltartan counterpart, its frequency is minimal as it is only mentioned once in the former and twice in the latter.[10] It is therefore almost redundant in her folklore collections.

[10] In "Herb-Healing," Gregory only writes "a herb" once when she mentions "a Galway woman" who "was delicate one time myself, and I lost my walk; and one of the neighbours told my mother it wasn't myself that was there" but her mother, however, said that "she'd soon find that out; for she'd tell me she was going to get a herb that would cure me; and if it was myself, I'd want it; but if it was another, I'd be against it" (*Poets and Dreamers* 118). In "Herbs, Charms, and Wise Women," a "*Slieve Echtge Woman*" tells Gregory about "Moyra Colum" who "was a great one for doing cures" and healed an injured horse as she "went into the field, and she picked a blade of a herb and put it to the horse's mouth and in

Gregory's movement from dismissing "a herb" to employing "an herb" reflects a wider movement in her works, from dismissing local Irish models to adopting and championing them.

* * *

It is possible that Gregory helped Yeats with his herbal knowledge, and that Yeats gleaned information about traditional medicine from Gregory, who had before learnt about healing plants from Ruane. Gregory creates the opportunity to mention an array of herbs in *The Pot of Broth*. In response to the tramp's question about the slanlus, Sibby replies, "No, indeed, I have none of that in the house" (*VPl* line 162). This opens a chasm that allows the tramp to ask another question involving herbs: "Or a bit of the Fearavan that was picked when the wind was from the north?" (lines 163–64). Again, this herb belongs in Gregory's list that she recorded from Ruane's lesson because "[t]his is the *Fearaban* (water-buttercup); and it's good for every bone of your body" (113). When Sibby again responds, "No, indeed, I'm sorry there's none," Gregory sees the opportunity to explain a third herb. The tramp asks, "Or a sprig of the Athair-talav, the father of herbs?" (lines 165–67). Like the other herbs that Gregory employed in the play, this one is also associated with revival, preservation, and longevity. Gregory dictates Ruane's words in "Herb-Healing":

> This is *Athair-talav*, the father of all herbs (wild camomile). This is very hard to pull; and when you go for it, you must have a black-handled knife. And whatever way the wind is when you begin to cut it, if it changes while you're cutting it, you'll lose your mind. And if you are paid for cutting it, you can do it when you like; but if not, *they* mightn't like it. I knew a woman was cutting at one time, and a voice, an enchanted voice, called out: "Don't cut that if you are not paid, or you'll be sorry." But if you put a bit of this with every other herb you drink, you'll live for ever. My grandmother used

one minute it got up well" (*Visions and Beliefs* 2: 16–17). In the same chapter, Gregory writes up an account by a man named James Mangan whose "mother learned to do a great many cures from a woman from the North" (2: 19). Interestingly, Gregory writes both "an herb" and "a herb" in the same short account as James Mangan says that "[f]or a swelling in the throat it's an herb would be used" but then states that "[t]here's a herb called *rif* in your own garden is good for cures" (2: 19). This indicates that Gregory heard the "herb" being preceded by both the indefinite articles "a" and "an."

> to put a bit with everything she took, and she lived to be over a hundred. (*Poets and Dreamers* 113)

It is fascinating that the three herbs that Gregory chooses to feature in *The Pot of Broth* are associated with preservation and revival. Ruane dictates that the slanlus can "bring back the dead," the fearavan is "good for every bone" in the body, and the athair-talav is propitious for longevity as her grandmother used this herb "with everything she took, and she lived to be over a hundred" (112, 113).

As with the fearavan in the play, Gregory reports other accounts that mention the wind in relation to gathering herbs. The fearavan, which is "good for every bone of your body," correlates with "the green herbs that cover her [Ruane's] grave" of which "there are some that are 'good for every bone in the body,' and that are 'very good for a sore heart'" (*Poets and Dreamers* 113, 120). The tramp identifies the fearavan herb as being "picked when the wind was from the north?" (lines 163–64). For the athair-talav, too, Ruane says that "whatever way the wind is when you begin to cut it, if it changes while you're cutting it, you'll lose your mind" (Gregory, *Poets and Dreamers* 113). One of Gregory's neighbours, later identified as Mrs. Quaid in "Herbs, Charms, and Wise Women," attaches the same precaution to the "*slanugad* (rib-grass)" when she warns, "[M]ind would the wind change when you are pulling it or your head will be gone" (*Visions and Beliefs* 2: 8). In "Herbs, Charms, and Wise Women," Gregory speaks to a woman named Mrs. Ward, who similarly says that "[a]s to the *lus-mor*, whatever way the wind is blowing when you begin to cut it, if it changes while you're cutting it, you'll lose your mind" (2: 9). The superstitious theory behind this folk belief is explained in "Herb-Healing" when an "old man," later recognised as "*Old Heffernan*" in "Herbs, Charms, and Wise Women," tells Gregory that he had "a lump on the thigh one time, and my father went to him [the herb-doctor Connolly/Conolly], and he gave him an herb for it; but he told him not to come into the house by the door the wind would be blowing in at" because "[t]hey thought it was the evil I had—that is given by *them* by a touch; and that is why he said about the wind; for if it was the evil there would be a worm in it, and if it smelled the herb that was brought in at the door, it might change to another place" (*Poets and Dreamers* 115–16; *Visions and Beliefs* 2: 11–12). The pot of broth is part of the silliness and trickery and the tramp's attempt to fool and beguile the couple, but the cautiousness and concern with which people discussed herbs in the Irish countryside means that the comedy comes from a division between what is said and what is done. What is said sounds like herbal lore that is serious and connotes status; what is done is the tramp putting onions and cabbage in a pot.

As to why people believed that the wind had to be blowing from a northern direction, this is most likely explained in Gregory's notes at the end of *Visions and Beliefs* as she clarifies that "north" does not refer to a geographical location such as Ulster but rather "[t]he North where the old Celtic other world was thought to lie is the quarter of spells and faeries" (2: 343). She also writes, "A woman from the North would probably be a faery woman or at any rate a 'knowledgeable' woman, one who was 'in the faeries' and certainly not necessarily at all a woman from Ulster" (2: 343). Gregory deliberately placed specific knowledge, including the fearavan and the perceived risk of psychological illness if it was gathered incorrectly, in the mouth of a tramp in accordance with her claim in *The Kiltartan Poetry Book: Prose Translations from the Irish* (1919) that she found "poetic emotion ... among farmers and potato diggers and old men in workhouses and beggars at my own door" (11). Gregory had gathered herbal knowledge from the rural people of Ireland, and she was not prepared to disregard or treat this lightly in *The Pot of Broth.*

The tramp's eventual use of "*cabbage and onions*" is certainly not medicinal (line 171). As "[t]here's plenty of it [slanlus] by the hedge," Sibby's husband John offers to "go out and get it" for the tramp (lines 168–69). However, the tramp insists that "those leaves beside me will do well enough" and "[*h*]*e takes a couple of good handfuls of the cabbage and onions and puts them in*" (lines 170–71). Leaves also feature in Gregory's chapter as she mentions a person named Farrell, who reports that "[t]he *Bainne bo blathan* (primrose) is good for the headache, if you put the leaves of it on your head" (*Poets and Dreamers* 116). However, through clearly identifying the "leaves" as vegetables, Gregory ensures that they cannot be mistaken for anything medicinal. It is highly likely that, in order to include herbal language in *The Pot of Broth*, Gregory referred back to "Herb-healing," a chapter that she dated and thus probably wrote in 1900 and then published just two years before this play in 1902. Her encounters with the rural Irish people would have been fresh in her mind, and the stories, accounts, and experiences that they imparted to her flowered in *The Pot of Broth.*

* * *

The pot, the centrepiece of the play alongside the broth and the stone, has social and poetical associations. Early in the play, there is a song that concentrates on both broth and the pot that holds it, and it was found by Gregory:

> There's broth in the pot for you, old man,
> There's broth in the pot for you, old man,
> There's cabbage for me
> And broth for you,
> And beef for Jack the journeyman.
>
> I wish you were dead, my gay old man,
> I wish you were dead, my gay old man,
> I wish you were dead
> And a stone at your head,
> So as I'd marry poor Jack the journeyman. (lines 61–70)

Visually, both stanzas are set out in the shape of a pot resting on the stove, and the lyric poem has therefore metamorphosed from a song that is heard to a concrete poem that can be seen. As Gregory first heard this song and wrote it down, it is likely that her and Yeats then set it out.

The first stanza is about the broth in the pot; the second stanza mentions a stone in the form of a grave. Whilst Gregory found the song on her folkloric travels, it was Yeats who then also took great interest in it. Pethica writes, "His only note for the play in early printings focuses exclusively on 'There's Broth in the Pot' — the first song the Tramp sings — describing it as 'taken down from an old woman known as Cracked Mary, who wanders about the plain of Aidhne, and who sometimes sees unearthly riders on white horses coming through stony fields to her hovel door in the night time'" (*Collaborative One-Act Plays* xlvi; *VPl* 254). Pethica confirms, "The unnamed collector was in fact Lady Gregory, who had recorded Cracked Mary's words in January 1899" (xlvi-xlvii; *Lady Gregory's Diaries* 201). The broth and the stone, both mentioned in the song, are the bread and butter of the simple play and therefore this song may have been the muse for *The Pot of Broth*.

Gregory recorded this song, which may have impacted the construction of the collaborative play, in a diary entry that was dated on 11 January 1899:

> "I wish you were dead my dear old man
> I wish you were dead & the sod on your head

> And I'd marry poor Jack the journeyman —
> There's broth in the pot for you old man
> There's broth for me & cabbage for you
> & beef for Jack the journeyman" — (*Lady Gregory's Diaries* 201)

The "broth" and "pot" and "*cabbage*" and "beef" are words that are carried into the play in so far as there is "a stone that could make broth," "a pot with a drop of boiling water in it," the "*cabbage and onions*," and the tramp's claim that the stone "is better than beef and mutton, and currant cakes and sacks of flour" (*VPl* lines 145, 149–50, 171, 129–30). According to Pethica, "She or Yeats would find a prior source for the song in an eighteenth-century volume of Scottish ballads" that is named *Ancient and Modern Scottish Songs, Heroic Ballads, Etc. Collected from Memory, Tradition, and Ancient Authors* (1776) in which this song is titled "I wiſh that you were dead, Goodman" (*Collaborative One-Act Plays* xlvii; *Scottish Songs* 2: 207–08). In the early typescript for *The Pot of Broth*, Gregory "typed" a "transcription" of this song (Pethica xlvii). As the song in the Scottish anthology is set out like a typical poem, and Gregory firstly wrote it down by listening to the words, the visual representation of the song has been added by Yeats and Gregory.

Yeats and Gregory's *The Pot of Broth* echoes the pots that were used in the Great Irish Famine, which spanned from 1845 to 1852. The "good drop of broth or a bit of stirabout, or a drop of poteen itself" that the tramp claims can be the result of placing the stone "down in a pot with a drop of water" and then proceeding to "stir it awhile" (lines 194–97). The Choctaw tribe, a group of Native American people who lived in Oklahoma, generously donated approximately $710 to the Irish people to help them survive the Famine (Howe and Kirwan xxvii). This enabled the provision of communal pots that were used in the Famine to nourish and feed the mass victims. These pots "are often colloquially known as famine pots" that were "[d]esigned to hold sufficient food to cater for a large number of people at one time" and "were often provided and stocked by charitable foundations and groups" (Howe and Kirwan xxxii). In their book *Famine Pots: The Choctaw-Irish Gift Exchange, 1847-Present* (2020), LeAnne Howe and Padraig Kirwan confirm that these famine pots "were often all that stood between life and death" (xxxii). However, they are also aware that "[t]hey have a somewhat controversial place in history too; many commentators have accused religious missionaries of providing soup in return for promises of conversion" and that "[o]thers point out that these pots were sometimes placed at the workhouses that tenant farmers were herded towards in some famine-stricken parts of Ireland" (Howe and Kirwan xxxii). Howe and Kirwan conclude, "However we interpret the story of these pots, the fact remains that their very existence reminds us of strife and endurance, hunger and charity, death and survival, want and plenty" (xxxii). Whilst Howe and Kirwan highlight that these pots "are a powerful emblem of the Great Famine," it is also plausible that they encompass the themes inherent in Yeats and Gregory's *The Pot of Broth* (xxxii).

When there was no food to place in the pot, it is possible that a stone would be placed in the pot to feign cooking to trick the mind into thinking that the stomach is full as this is a hunger-delaying technique employed in hunger crises such as the Madagascar Famine of 2021. On 11 November 2021, a six-year-old child in Madagascar named Sambeanake said that "[*w*]*e pretend to cook rice with soil and sand, stones as meat*" and "[*w*]*e also pretend to eat that good meal*" (Cook, et al., "Madagascar"). This mirrors the aspect of the tramp's trickery that involves placing the stone in the pot with the illusion that "you'll have the thing you were wanting ready before you" (lines 197–98). In the Famine, when there were no ingredients for soup, poor substitutes from the environment would have gone into the pot. For example, in *Continuity and Change in Irish Poetry, 1966–2010* (2012), Eric Falci states that "many of the starving took to eating grass as the only form of food available, and images of faces marked by a green grass-stain are part of the cultural memory of the Famine" (179). This pot became an important symbol for the victims of the Irish Famine. In *A History of Ireland in 100 Objects* (2013), Fintan O'Toole states, "These pots became a talisman of survival" (247). Estyn Evans writes that the sufferers "clung to the pot when all else was gone" (qtd. in O'Toole 247). Even though the famine pots were often empty or otherwise filled with grass or other countryside materials that could not sustain the body, the pot itself was a source of hope and a chance at life for the hungry. The play contains herbal healing, someone trying to steal a pot, and someone boiling a stone. Tragedy is not far beneath the comedic surface. Even though the play is a comedy, somehow the ghost of the Famine is heard in it.

In *The Pot of Broth*, the tramp also values the cooking pot as his desire develops from only wanting "the loan of a pot" to asking Sibby if he can keep the pot even though his initial aim was to be given food (line 149). He claims that "[t]he world and all wouldn't buy it, ma'am," but then says that "[t]he whole world wouldn't coax it out of me except maybe for one thing ... [*looks depressed*]" and that "[n]ow I think of it, there's only one reason I might think of parting with it at all" (lines 294, 299–302; ellipsis in source). Sibby "*eagerly*" asks, "What reason is that?" and this is met with the following response:

> TRAMP. It's a misfortune that overtakes me, ma'am, every time I make an attempt to keep a pot of my own to boil it in, and I don't like to be always under a compliment to the neighbours, asking the loan of one. But whatever way it is, I never can keep a pot with me. I had a right to ask one of the little man that gave me the stone. The last one I bought got the bottom burned out of it one night I was giving a hand to a friend that keeps a still, and the one before that I hid under a bush one time I was going into Ennis for the night, and some boys in the town dreamed about it and went looking for treasure in it, and they found nothing but eggshells, but they brought it away for all that. And another one ...
>
> SIBBY. Give me the loan of the stone itself, and I'll engage I'll keep a pot for it.... Wait now till I'll make some offer to you.... (lines 303–21; ellipses in source)

As pots placed on the fire were often the centrepiece of the Irish kitchen, so are the themes of the play centred around the famine pot. There are patterns that involve the pot being accidentally destroyed, the pot being taken from someone else, and other problems surrounding the retention of the pot. The tramp reveals that three pots in total have been taken from him by some form of "misfortune that overtakes me" (line 304). This highlights the fragility of these highly sought-after pots and their recognised importance in Ireland. A line from the song "Paistin Finn" intensifies the echoes of the Irish Famine even more: "And I am shrunken to skin and bone" (line 251). At the resolution, the tramp addresses Sibby and says that "as you were so kind, and for the sake of the good treatment you gave me, I'll ask nothing at all for it" and "[h]ere it is for you and welcome, and that you may live long to use it!" (lines 331–35). This is an ironic expression as the tramp takes all their food, which impedes survival. Like the Famine victims, Sibby and John are left clinging to their empty famine pot when their food has been taken away. Though it is never openly addressed in the play, the Great Famine haunts its action and language.

* * *

For Gregory, herbs had a metaphorical significance and she used them to get to the root of Ireland's illnesses. She associated herbs with the Irish countryside and the soil from which they grew; she realised that there was a deeper meaning beneath the surface. Gregory came across this hidden meaning and the phrase "an herb" when she translated Douglas Hyde's "An Craoibhin Complains Because He is a Poet," a poem about hunger and Irish identity, for *Poets and Dreamers*:

> It's my grief that I am of the race of the poets;
> It would be better for me to be a high rock,
> Or a stone or a tree or an herb or a flower
> Or anything at all, but the thing that I am. (79)

Hyde presents the herb as not a literal medicine to *use* but as something *to be* and to imitate. In the Irish countryside, herbs were used to revive the sick; Hyde similarly wanted to revive the Irish language, ailing due to English colonial rule, back to full health. This poem, lamenting a threatened Irish identity, was described by Gregory as having been written "in the form of a little folk-song" that "expresses the thought of the idealist of all time, that makes him [Hyde] cry, as one of the oldest of the poets cried long ago, 'Mine heritage is unto me as a speckled bird; the birds round about are against her'" (*Poets and Dreamers* 78). Gregory analysed, "The sympathy of the moods of nature with the moods of man is a traditional heritage that has come to us through the poets, from the old time when the three great waves of the sea answered to a cry of distress in Ireland, or when, as in Israel, the land mourned and the herbs of every field withered, for the wickedness of them that dwelt therein" (*Poets and Dreamers* 79). Gregory was not only aware of the presence of herbs in the rural landscape, where they were used as medicine, but she also witnessed them crop up in Revival-era literature.

Yeats and Gregory may have used one of Hyde's poems as a model for Cathleen Ni Houlihan's monologue that lists the sacrifices for Ireland. In *Poets and Dreamers*, Gregory introduces this poem with the introduction: "Here is a fine vision of a battle-field" (85). Hyde writes that "[t]he time I think of the cause of Ireland," it is then that "[m]y heart is torn within me" (85). He laments the deceased Irishmen who fought for Ireland yet were "[h]idden under grass, or under tall herbs" and were "[f]ar from friends or help or friendship" and there was "[n]ot a child or a wife near them" (85). He also sympathises with the "many a married woman" who is "[w]ithout her comrade, without a father for her child tonight" (86). This sacrificial overtone is carried into Cathleen's prophecy that "[m]any that are red-cheeked now will be pale-cheeked," that "many a good plan will be broken," and that "many a child will be born and there will be no father at its christening to give it a name" (lines 303, 306, 308–09). Hyde's poem mentions herbs that cover the bodies, yet Yeats and Gregory's version put reviving herbs into practice as the bearers of these sacrifices are presented as being "remembered," "alive," "speaking," and heard "for ever" (lines 313–16). Similarly, in Yeats's *The King's Threshold* (1904), the poet Seanchan is starved and represents a new era of emotions of the heart. This is another play that involves individual loss for a collective cause because a poet starves to death as a political stand against a king that would not listen to him about the importance of art for art's sake.

In an early draft of *Cathleen Ni Houlihan* (1902), soup plays a part in the drama but is excised in later versions. This "draft of *Cathleen ni Houlihan*" is "in Lady Gregory's hand, on leaves loosely gathered in the separated covers of a terracotta-colored 'penny' exercise book" (Pethica, *Collaborative One-Act Plays* xiii). On the twenty-first page, there is "a leaf torn from a bifolium of light blue Coole Park stationery" and "[t]he material drafted on this page has been deleted with three vertical strokes in black ink and one in orange pencil" (Pethica xiii). In this draft, a line was written for Michael or another one of the characters in the cottage: "*Will you have a drink of milk [& a bit] & a [bowl] bit of the soup -?*" (45). Cathleen Ni Houlihan, however, replies that "[*t*]*he time is not come for eating & drinking -*" (45). Food is outright rejected in this play where there is initially money and costly clothes. Cathleen brings with her a harsher but more idealistic world.

The tramp in *The Pot of Broth*, like Cathleen Ni Houlihan, disturbs the scene. Yeats and Gregory had very different ideas about what characters who intervene in the action and overturn a settled order look like. In relation to the poet Raftery in *The Marriage* and the ragged man in *The Rising of the Moon*, Pethica poses an argument about Gregory and her artist-healers in the introduction to his *Collaborative One-Act Plays*:

> In Lady Gregory's plays, the artist-disturber is invariably a healer who is able to effect some form of beneficial influence in the world of ordinary materiality, and who is able to promote compromise, even if only briefly, between the competing demands of idealism and the needs of the ordinary world: her early plays *The Marriage* (1902) and *The Rising of the Moon* (1903) are paradigmatic. A core vision of the artist as a healer who comes to repair the social

> economy or to inspire others, but who then typically withdraws unobtrusively, would underpin her principal work as a dramatist, and also inform her optimistic core conception of the theater movement as a venue in which artists such as Yeats, herself, and others might model beneficial social and political change for Ireland. In Yeats's work, by contrast, the visionary/disturber invariably generates conflict, loss, or political rupture by demanding complete commitment to an ideal that calls for decisive and often violent transformation or overthrow of ordinary reality. (lvi–lvii)

Unlike Yeats, Gregory casts gentle yet powerful healers into her plays who carry moral messages that motivate positive change at both the individual and societal level; she views healers and healing as the medicators and medicines that will construct a new and peaceful place in which to live and write.

In *The Marriage*, the poet Raftery is disguised as a blind fiddler. Martin and Mary, a newlywed couple, welcome him into their new home and provide him with food as "it is likely there is hunger on you" (*Poets and Dreamers* 220). Unaware of his true identity as Raftery, who is described by Mary as being recently deceased following "his sickness at some place near Killeenan," the couple's dual hospitality is rewarded as Raftery then heals their financial difficulties at a communal and societal level (217). When Raftery reveals who he is, Mary says that "I see no sign of sickness on you now" and he replies that "I am well, I am well now, the Lord be praised for it" (223–24). Raftery tells the couple to "open the door wide, and let the blessing of God come in on you" (222). He "*takes up his fiddle and begins to play on it*" and then appeared the "[l]ittle boys that came to listen to [him]" (222). Outside the cottage, there are also "carts coming home from the fair" and Raftery asks the boys to "stop the people; tell them they must come in" and "there will be as fine a dance as ever they saw" (223). He adds that "they must all give a present to the man and woman that are newly married" (223). Raftery gives Mary his gift of a "*plate of money*," which was the sum of the neighbours' contributions for his music (234). He says, "Take that and my seven hundred blessings along with it, and that you may be as well as I wish you to the end of life and time" and "[c]ount the money now, and see what the neighbours did for you" (234). Raftery inconspicuously exits the scene at the resolution and Martin asks a young man if he had seen "a blind fiddler going out the door—the poet Raftery?" (235). The young man replies, "I did not; but I stood by his grave at Killeenan three days ago" (235). This time frame echoes Jesus's resurrection from the dead after three days. The final line, spoken by Martin, confirms Raftery's role in the play as "a man sent by God" for societal healing in the form of the promotion of widespread generosity (235).

In the political play *The Rising of the Moon*, a ragged man rekindles a sergeant's "great spirit" for Irish independence, a flame that had been dampened by his role in the Royal Irish Constabulary (148). The play is set at the "[*s*]*ide of a quay in a seaport town*," where a sergeant is "mind[ing] this place" and is on the lookout for a man who had "broke[n] out of goal" (*Selected Plays* 143, 144). A ragged man, who is this wanted prisoner and is disguised as "Jimmy Walsh, a ballad-singer," enters the scene and tells the sergeant about "the man you're waiting for" (144, 146). Probably scaremongering rather than speaking truth, he suggests that the escaped prisoner killed "a poor man in our place, a sergeant from Ballyvaughan... with a lump of stone" (146). As with the stone in *The Pot of Broth*, Gregory is perhaps using this same prop as a tool of trickery for the ragged man's anecdotes, which are possibly crafted to frighten the sergeant who himself admits that "[y]ou made me feel a bit queer with the way you talked" (147). This allows the ragged man to remind him that "it was with the people you were, and not with the law you were, when you were a young man" and prompts the sergeant to remember that "I had a great spirit in those days" (149, 148). At the resolution, the sergeant sacrifices the "hundred pounds reward" by letting the ragged man escape, thus denying materialism in favour of Irish freedom (151). Through the ragged man, who refers to a time when "the small rise up and the big fall down" and "when we all change places at the Rising (*waves his hand and disappears*) of the Moon," Gregory speaks of a non-violent and political ideal (151).

Prior to mentioning *The Marriage* and *The Rising of the Moon*, which he views as "paradigmatic" for including "a healer who is able to effect some form of beneficial influence in the world of ordinary materiality," Pethica mentions a Yeats-Gregory collaboration that "brought essential differences between the two writers into play" (*Collaborative One-Act Plays* lvi). *The Travelling Man*, published in 1905, is a miracle play about "a Christ figure who helps a homeless woman to find shelter and safety, and whose subsequent return reminds her of her spiritual obligations" (Pethica lv). At the exposition, the homeless woman describes Jesus Christ as "a very tall man, the best I ever saw" and "bright and shining" (*Selected*

Plays 22).[11] Jesus tells the woman that "I will come to see you some other time" and "do not shut up your heart in the things I give you … but have a welcome before me" (22).[12] When Jesus returns to the house, the woman does not look past His appearance as a travelling man and does not welcome Him. She later regrets her inhospitality when her child tells her that, after the mother told Him to leave the house, He was "walking on the water" and she realises that her visitor was "the King of the World" (28). Pethica writes that Yeats's and Gregory's "inability to work together productively on the project was in the end not merely a result simply of the tension between Lady Gregory's orthodox Christianity and Yeats's heterodox 'Pagan' tendencies, or, say, between her penchant for the realist method and his preference for symbolism, but was at root also a consequence of their very different conceptions of the functions of art itself" (*Collaborative One-Act Plays* lvi). Communicated through the play, Gregory's healing message is to see Jesus in all people and take care of our neighbours, which are moral duties that she was passionate about in her own life.

The visitor/disturber in *The Pot of Broth* follows the Yeatsian model. He pretends to possess a magical stone that can make "a good drop of broth or a bit of stirabout, or a drop of poteen itself" (lines 194–96). Near the outset of the play, when the tramp says that "I know what I'll do, I know what the tinker did with a stone," this is an allusion to a well-known story about this exact pretence (lines 56–57). Thought to originate from a French folk narrative written in 1720, and adapted by different authors from then on, the storyline of a beggar who subtly persuades people to contribute to his broth travelled across Europe (Rubel).[13] This narrative

[11] Gregory read the Bible throughout her life; of course, she would have known about Jesus Christ, who is the Divine Physician, and she would have read the accounts of His healings.

[12] Gregory's inspiration for writing *The Travelling Man* may have emerged from the words of a basket maker, which she encountered in an experience that she recorded in her diary on 28 June 1898: "I took Jack Ford & Daly to the wood for spruce trees they wanted for their haycocks — Daly found one he thought wd [abbreviation for 'would'] do, but when guiding me to see it, he could not come across it again — & J. F. called out 'has it gone astray on you!' — The basket maker says: May the Lord Jesus be a travelling man at the end of the universe to lead you straight to [H]eaven —" (*Lady Gregory's Diaries* 188).

[13] In his webpage "History of the Stone Soup Folktale from 1720 to Now," William Rubel traces the first publication of this story back to a French journalist named Madame de Noyer whose "Soupe au Caillou" was published in a collection of letters titled *Lettres Historiques et Galantes, De Deux Dames de Condition, dont l'une étoit à Paris, et l'autre en Province* in

circulated in Ireland, as evident in informant Mrs. Gerety's "A Funny Story" in *The Schools' Manuscript Collection* (*NFCS*) in which "a poor man came to the door of a rich man and asked for something to eat as he was very hungry" (85).[14] Dismissed by the wealthy man, the poor man "came upon a heap of stones and he picked up one and said I know what I will do I will make stone soup" and "the woman of the house" next door "gave him the pot with the water & he put the stone in it" (85, 86). Then, "[a]fter some time he asked her would she give him, a little bit of butter" and "[s]he gave him a piece of butter about the size of an egg" as well as "an onion" and "a good cut of bread to eat with the stone soup, so the poor man satisfied his hunger" (86). Although Gregory had the tools to make the tramp a healer, she could not employ them for a disturber. Instead, she had no choice but to leave them out of the pot and the drama; she instead continued to gather herbs and fruits and even stones that would be used in her own play in 1916.

* * *

The Golden Apple (1916), too, is a children's play that hints at Gregory's early interest in herbal medicine through a search for a healing apple. It explores the themes of ageing, death, medical cures, the elixir of life, and the potential for renewal. In it, the King of Ireland is ill and so his son Rury and the steward Simon embark upon a quest to find "the golden apple that will cure any sickness at all or any wound" (216; act 3, sc. 1). After much difficulty in finding the apple, involving encounters with a witch and an imprisoned princess and a giant and a scheming doctor, both Rury and Simon successfully bring the cure to the King who then becomes a younger and healthier version of himself. In this drama, the doctor diagnoses the giant Fatach Mor with having "swallowed a water-worm or an

1720. Subsequent versions include: Phillipe Barbe's "La Soupe au Caillou" in *Fables et Contes Philosophiques* (1771), Robert Moser's first publication of this narrative in the English language in *The European Magazine, and London Review* (1806), an adaptation printed in *The American Magazine of Wit* (1808) by a writer who uses the pseudonym The Judge of Conviviality, and an Irish version of this folk story that was published in *Irish Wit, or Post-Chaise Companion* in 1812 by a writer disguised by the pseudonym Momus Broadgrin (Rubel).

[14] *NFCS* 0751: 85–86; Mrs. Gerety (32), Gorteenclareen, County Longford. Collector: Teresa Gerety, Gurteen, Ballymahon [school], Gorteenclareen, County Longford. 22 November 1937–19 December 1938. Teacher: T. Ó. Murchadha.

eel" (250; act 2, sc. 2). This is inspired by Gregory's "Herb Healing" chapter, where she writes about a person who was suffering with this same ailment:

> "Sea-grass" is sometimes useful as a natural and sometimes as an occult cure. One who has tried it and other herbs, says: "Indeed the porter did me good, and good that I'd hardly like to tell you, not to make a scandal. Did I drink too much of it? Not at all. But this long time I am feeling a worm in my side that is as big as an eel, and there's more of them in it than that. And I was told to put sea-grass to it; and I put it to the side the other day; and whether it was that or the porter I don't know, but there's some of them gone out of it.["] (*Poets and Dreamers* 118–19)

Gregory also draws upon mythological medical material as well as herbal remedies. The giant's wife states, "There is some doctors who can recognise what sickness is on a man by the smoke they see going out of the chimney of his house" (249–50; act 2, sc. 2). This is a cross-reference to medical information in Gregory's *Cuchulain of Muirthemne*: "Now, Fingan was the greatest physician in all Ireland, and it was said of him that he could tell what a person's sickness was by looking at the smoke of the house he was in" (246). The giant's wife adds another inaccurate theory: "I knew of one could tell it [the sickness] by measuring you" (250; act 2, sc. 2). This is similar to the giant's earlier comment that "[t]here is more room for the pain to work by reason of the height of my body and the length there is in my limbs" (235; act 1, sc. 4). Gregory alluded to this diagnostic tool in the later "Herbs, Charms, and Wise Women," a chapter in the second series of *Visions and Beliefs in the West of Ireland*, in which "[*a*] *Slieve Echtge Woman*" reports that "[t]here's one woman I knew used to take a bit of tape when you'd go to her, and she'd measure it over her thumb like this; and when she had it measured she'd know what was the matter with you" (2: 16, 18).[15] Gregory's bank of medicinal knowledge, collected in the long term from books and people and places, served her well in terms of mixing remedies for her neighbourhood and writing cures into her work.

[15] Yeats also knew about the use of measuring as a diagnostic tool as, in his essay "The Queen and the Fool" (1901), he writes that there is "an old woman who lives in the Bog of Kiltartan, and is very poor" who said that "[t]here was an old man I knew long ago, he had a tape, and he could tell what diseases you had with measuring you" (*Mythologies* 75).

There are numerous references to healing in *The Golden Apple*, most of which emanate from the mouths of the steward Simon, the giant's wife and, of course, the doctor with his metaphorical "coat of healing" (236; act 1, sc. 4). Addressing Fatach Mor, the giant's wife says, "My joy go with you in a bottle of moss, and if you never come back you'll be no great loss!" (236; act 1, sc. 4). As moss is a preservative herb, the giant's wife probably said this in order to prolong her joy that she has figuratively given to Fatach Mor. The "ball of flax" that is "[t]wisted … on a crooked holly stick" is another allusion to "Herb-Healing" (238; act 1, sc. 4). Gregory writes down Ruane's assertion that "[t]here is something in flax, for no priest would anoint you without a bit of tow" as well as other accounts of the protective properties of flax:

> And a neighbour of hers confirms this, and says: "There's something in green flax, I know; for my mother often told me about one night she was spinning flax before she was married, and she was up late. And a man of the fairies came in—she had no right to be sitting up so late: they don't like that—and he told her it was time to go to bed; for he wanted to kill her, and he couldn't touch her while she was handling the flax....["] (*Poets and Dreamers* 119–20)

Therefore, "every time he'd tell her to go to bed, she'd give him some answer, and she'd go on pulling a thread of the flax, or mending a broken one" until "at the crowing of the cock he'd have to go" and "she was safe" because the cockerel "is blessed" (120). Holly is also a traditional plant that has protective properties. *The Schools' Manuscript Collection* (*NFCS*) reports that, traditionally, the cure for "'[w]ild [f]ire' or [f]ever" was to "[h]ang holly over the door" ("Local Cures" 156).[16] Symbolic for protection, it was also used to make the St. Brigid's Cross, which is "a pinwheel made of river rushes, representing the eternal turning of the seasons back to spring" (Clark 62). Many of the herbs that Gregory includes in her play have shielding and defensive properties.

Gregory places more medical and mythological cures in the mouth of the Irish steward Simon than the doctor, a figure that is depicted as "hav[ing] knowledge enough to take your money, giving your sickness every name longer than another" (236; act 1; sc. 4). Whilst Simon aims to

[16] *NFCS* 0800: 156; Clonbulloge [school], Clonbulloge, County Offaly, 20 June 1938–27 June 1938. Teacher: A. Fitzgerald.

cure the King with "hot stones," a remedy grounded in traditional Irish medicine, the doctor instead references mythology as well as medicine (224; act 1, sc. 2). Although the doctor's "sheepskin" may have given the King warmth and encouraged recovery, it is also similar to the magical pigskin in "The Sons of Tuireann" in *Gods and Fighting Men* (1904) (225; act 1, sc. 2). In this narrative, "Brian, one of the sons of Tuireann" defeated a man in battle and "then he kept a hold of the [pig] skin and put it about himself" (26, 40). In total, the three Tuireann sons affirmed, "We are well off when we have the apples and the skin" (40). Addressing Simon in *The Golden Apple*, Muireann says, "You to have had the smallest wound in the world, he [Rury] would have searched out herbs of healing to put round about you" and questions, "Why did it fail you to go search the whole face of the world for a cure for the King's son?" (260; act 2, sc. 3). The maintenance of health is one of the thematic mainstays of the play.

Gregory writes, "Old Bridget Ruane will not do any more cures by charms or by simples, or 'bring children home to the world' any more" because "she died last winter; and we may be sure that among the green herbs that cover her grave, there are some that are 'good for every bone in the body,' and that are 'very good for a sore heart'" (*Poets and Dreamers* 120). This alludes to Míach in "The Reign of Bres" in *Gods and Fighting Men*. When he dies, we are told that "herbs grew up from his grave, to the number of his joints and sinews, three hundred and sixty-five" (Gregory 13). In this way, Gregory compares Ruane to a mythological hero.

Gregory's "Herb-Healing" became a handbook for her plays and, after Ruane's death, she continued to accumulate knowledge about traditional medicine, which she would go on to publish in *Visions and Beliefs* in 1920, a more substantial folklore collection that highlights her development in medicine since 1900. Gregory's twenty-year span between "Herb-Healing" and *Visions and Beliefs* is a strictly medical transformation period from 1900 to 1920. Gregory's first chapter about Ruane began her medico-literary career and inspired her fictional works, such as *The Golden Apple*, which is bookended by her larger folklore collection in 1920.

* * *

At the same time as Lady Gregory was innovating a new literary language based on her locality in the west of Ireland, she created a symbolic language of healing herbs. Her folklore collections, specifically in relation to herbs, formed a foundation for her entire literary career and gave her a form of communication that could reach a universal audience. Whilst Gregory did not get a chance to fully root the herbs in *The Pot of Broth*, due to the tramp not fitting into a healing role, she later planted the herbs in more suitable soil and was able to reap more benefits from her many years of collecting folklore. Her early collaborative works with Yeats gave her time to gather and think about how she would use the herbs in a solo work. By writing *Poets and Dreamers* and *Visions and Beliefs*, Gregory induced a delayed recognition for her herbalism teacher Ruane and brought her knowledge of healing and cures into the compass of the Irish Revival. Both Gregory and Yeats strived to benefit Ireland as a nation and the world. The way to communicate was not only through words: herbal salves might be an element in global salvation.

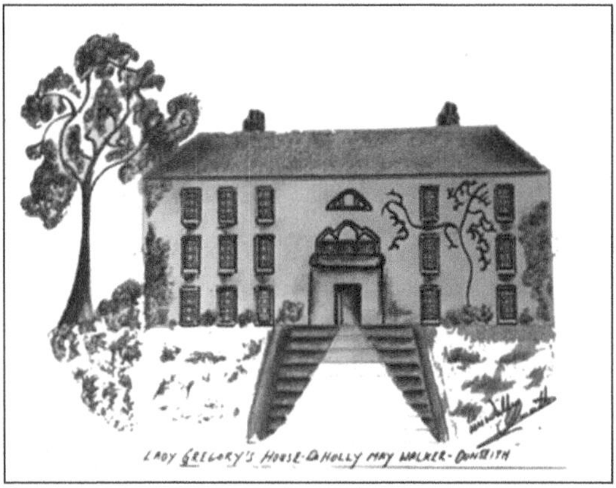

Lady Gregory's House

PART III

J. M. Synge: Wells, Wellness and Well-Being

CHAPTER 6

Synge and Congestion: The Respiratory System of the West

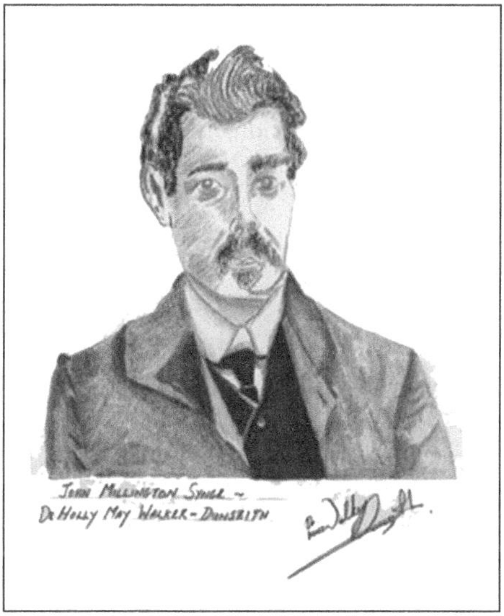

John Millington Synge

H. M. Walker-Dunseith, *Traditional Medicine in the Irish Literary Revival*, New Directions in Irish and Irish American Literature,
https://doi.org/10.1007/978-3-031-82459-3_6

It is no coincidence that Synge uses a *well* to explore his personal definition of *well*-being. In *The Well of the Saints* (1905), he employs "well" as a homonym to mean both the literal well and to describe good eyesight. Timmy says that "[t]here's a green ferny *well*, I'm told, behind of that place, and if you put a drop of the water out of it, on the eyes of a blind man, you'll make him see as *well* as any person is walking the world" (*CW* 3: 79; act 1; emphases added).[1] Here, Synge distinguishes between "a miraculous spring of water" with "medicinal properties" and "well-being" and "welfare" ("Well"; *OED*).[2] For Synge, the physical body of the well is a microcosm for the wider metaphysical concept of wellness.

Synge deploys the word "well-being" in an intriguing context in his travel essay "From Galway to Gorumna" in his collection *In Wicklow, West Kerry and Connemara* (1911).[3] He uses this word in an ambiguous context in a description of a rural place in the west:

> One's first feeling as one comes back among these people and takes a place, so to speak, in this noisy procession of fishermen, farmers, and women, where nearly everyone is interesting and attractive, is a dread of any reform that would tend to lessen their individuality rather than any very real hope of improving their well-being. (*CW* 2: 286)[4]

At the beginning of the twentieth century, there was much philosophical debate over "well-being" as a subjective concept that is person-centred rather than an objective truth.[5] Synge is more attracted by subjective measures of wellness and this is reflected in his play when the Doul couple are "choosing a wilful blindness" (143; act 3). The blind characters use their blind state to "be having an easy time with no trouble to live, and we

[1] Unless otherwise stated, the quotations for Synge's plays are taken from his *Collected Works, Volume III: Plays, Book I* (1968), edited by Ann Saddlemyer.

[2] At the time that Synge was writing in the early twentieth century, according to the anecdotal evidence provided by *Google Books Ngram Viewer*, there was an increase in the written usage of the word "well-being," which means, "[w]ith reference to a person or community: the state of being healthy, happy, or prosperous; physical, psychological, or moral welfare" ("well-being"; Orwant and Brockman; *OED*).

[3] Following serial publications, this essay was first published in book format in the fourth volume of *The Works of John M. Synge* titled *In Wicklow, In West Kerry, In the Congested Districts and Under Ether* (1910).

[4] Unless otherwise declared, the quotations for Synge's prose are taken from his *Collected Works, Volume II: Prose* (1982), edited by Alan Price.

[5] See Guy Fletcher's *The Routledge Handbook of Philosophy of Well-Being* (2017).

getting half-pence on the road" (143; act 3). Martin Doul says that Timmy, a hard-working blacksmith, is "sneezing and sweating since the dawn of day" (109; act 2). This contrasts with Martin Doul who is "after idling, and blathering, to this hour from the dawn of day" (107; act 2). Martin realises that he cannot be forced into work if he is disabled when he says that "it's more [money] I got a while since, and I sitting blinded in Grianan, than I get in this place, working hard, and destroying myself, the length of the day" (103; act 2). Synge was caught in the middle of contemporary well-being philosophies and ethics that looked at decision-making based on selfishness and happiness rather than virtue and intrinsic goodness.[6] In his play, Synge makes his standpoint clear: the healing water from the well, a resource and objective good available to the community, is rejected by the blind couple who value their subjective *well*-being.

In 1891, the British government diagnosed congestion in rural Ireland and administered a treatment: they decided to establish the Congested Districts Board, which underwent action to alleviate hardship in remote areas and make the west of Ireland more economically sustainable. When politician Arthur James Balfour introduced the bill in the House of Commons that would set up the Congested Districts Board, he uses the term "well-being" in considering the landlords whom his bill disadvantaged.[7] In the "Purchase of Land and Congested Districts (Ireland) Bill" (24 March 1890), Balfour said, "I believe that in England and Scotland the landlord class are not only a valuable social element, but that they contribute materially to the well-being of two other classes of the community engaged in the cultivation of the soil" (Hansard par. 1697). The *First Annual Report of the Congested Districts Board for Ireland* (1893) provides information about the history and workings of the Congested Districts Board, particularly as it operated in the Aran Islands, claiming that "[i]n short, the Board's efforts are to be directed as regards agriculture, towards increasing the size of small holdings and towards improving live stock and methods of cultivation; and in the second place towards aiding and developing all industries, including fishing" and "it is quite

[6] For example: hedonism, which underpins utilitarianism, is "[t]he doctrine or theory of ethics in which pleasure is regarded as the chief good, or the proper end of action" ("Hedonism"; *OED*). However, a decision that is made to attain a happy outcome does not mean that it is morally right and intrinsically good; happiness is not a reliable moral indicator. For more information on well-being philosophies, see Guy Fletcher's *The Routledge Handbook of Philosophy of Well-Being* (2017).

[7] I am grateful to Alex Davis for making this point.

clear that our Board was constituted with a view to bringing about a gradual and lasting improvement in the poor districts in the West of Ireland and not for the immediate '*relief*' of exceptional distress" (5). Wellness and well-being do not appear to be considered in this document and "well" is used to reference an alleged "remedy" that caused harm to Ireland rather than health. Horace Plunkett, an agricultural reformer, wrote that "[a]s I was obliged, from the necessity of the case, to act without definite instructions it is well that I should state briefly the nature and scope of the inquiry which I had undertaken" and that "[t]he Board, I was aware, might or might not at some future time see fit to assist emigration" but "[o]ther remedies so far as practicable would be preferred" (43). Plunkett continues, "[a]t the same time in some districts the chief remedy would be 'amalgamation of holdings,' and this would involve migration or emigration" (43). The British government diagnosed congestion, and they seemed to believe that it was this supposed "congestion" that caused symptoms of exceptional distress. However, these rural districts were scarcely populated, and the number of people was decreasing over time.[8] Emigration, the supposed remedy of decongestion, was therefore unnecessary and not a cure at all but rather a curb that deprived the Irish people of their traditional working lives and their homeland itself. What is presented as health, an opportunity for Ireland to have rural areas that are like decongested and healthy lungs that are breathing well, might actually be fitness for exploitation.

Synge believed that the Congested Districts Board represented a one-size-fits-all modernity that made unique Irish places homogenous and took more from them than was being given. In *The Aran Islands* (1906), Synge writes, "Kilronan, the principal village on Aranmor, has been so much changed by the fishing industry, developed there by the Congested Districts Board, that it has now very little to distinguish it from any fishing village on the west coast of Ireland" (*CW* 2: 47). Ciara Breathnach, writing on the redevelopment of Kilronan and boat building, states that "[o]nly one boat was ordered from the Kilronan (on Inishmore, the largest of the Aran Islands) yard in 1906, which failed to produce it in time for the summer fishery, and the board had to buy a second-hand Scottish

[8] According to Arthur Wilson Fox's "Report ... upon the Poor Law Union of Westport (Mayo)" in the Royal Commission on Labour's *The Agricultural Labourer* (1893), "[f]rom 1851 and 1881 the population of the county of Mayo decreased from 274,199 to 245,212, or 10.66 per cent., and had further decreased in 1891 to 219,034, or 1.65 per cent" (4: 56).

vessel instead" and so "Kilronan closed in 1907 when three of the shipwrights emigrated to America" (103).[9] It appears that the traditional fishing practices were needlessly amputated from Kilronan as part of a project of modernisation; they were replaced with the mechanical limb of industry that, far from being original to Ireland, was outsourced from elsewhere and could be replicated anywhere.

The "Congested Districts Board" is a title that invites debate. The word "congested" means "[h]eaped together; accumulated" and a "congested district" is "an area of land of which the resources are inadequate to support its population" ("Congested"; *OED*). It is ironic because these districts were sometimes among the most sparsely populated places in Ireland, such as Kilronan and Connemara. Breathnach asserts that "'Congested' was a label applied to the western counties in 1882 in the first report of 'Mr Tuke's Fund,'" a scheme that assisted people in emigrating from Ireland (11). It seems that "congested" was calculated based on a flawed equation. In his article "The Congested Districts Board" (1941), Seán M. Ó Conchubhair argues that "[t]he term 'congested' is only correct when applied to the actual patches of unproductive land upon which the tenants were confined and from which they tried to eke out a bare existence" and "[i]f the population of the counties be regarded as a whole, it could not be considered congested when taking the county area into account" (477). Furthermore, in *The Modernisation of Irish Society, 1848–1918* (1989), Joseph Lee argues that "[t]he Board's promise … generally far exceeded its performance" (125). To Synge, the Board represented the imposition of an unwelcome standardisation.

The narrative of "congestion" made the west of Ireland a sick patient. The British government, like the Saint in Synge's play, could "cure" this sick patient through emigration—decongesting the countryside. Suddenly, in this narrative, the destruction of traditional ways of life could be reimagined as beneficent healing. This relates to the characters in Synge's *The Well of the Saints*, a play whereby a blind couple refuse a Saint's cure that could permanently restore their eyesight. The Saint says to the blind couple that "[s]o it's to the like of yourselves I do be going, who are wrinkled and poor, a thing rich men would hardly look at at all, but would throw a coin to or a crust of bread" (89; act 1). Here, Synge is irreverently and ironically linking the Saint to the Congested Districts Board. The

[9] See Ciara Breathnach's *The Congested Districts Board of Ireland, 1891–1923: Poverty and Development in the West of Ireland* (2005).

British government identified what they perceived to be "wrinkled and poor" areas of Ireland and, instead of "throw[ing] a coin to or a crust of bread" to help the traditional Irish professions that were already in place, they used the Congested Districts Board to impose modernisation and emigration. The Congested Districts Board assessed the number of people in some rural Irish areas and then selected the districts that they believed did not work, like a congested lung that is failing. The British government appear to equate the word "congested" to what is now known as a GDP (Gross Domestic Product) model, which is a way to measure productivity by calculating how much money there is in the country dividing it by the number of inhabitants. This measure, though, has many blind spots. It does not reveal any data about happiness, working conditions, or how people find meaning in life. Synge seems to view money as a blunt instrument of measurement.

Synge uses the word "congested" to describe the weather in *In Wicklow, West Kerry and Connemara*. "The Oppression of the Hills" is a short commentary about life around the hills in County Wicklow and Synge's observation that "[a]mong the cottages that are scattered through the hills of County Wicklow I have met with many people who show in a singular way the influence of a particular locality" (*CW* 2: 209). Following his discussion about the "heavy rains," which are a regular occurrence for "every season," Synge writes:

> Then the clouds break, and there is a night of terrific storm from the south-west—all the larches that survive in these places are bowed and twisted towards the point where the sun rises in June—when the winds come down through the narrow glens with the *congested* whirl and roar of a torrent, breaking at times for sudden moments of silence that keep up the tension of the mind. (209; emphasis added).

It is interesting that Synge adopts the adjective "congested" to describe Wicklow, which is on the east coast and thus was not part of the Congested Districts; it is as if illness is a necessary part of the place. Here, "congested" is an adjective that describes the "whirl" of the weather that creates a crowded and overwhelmed atmosphere. It is interesting that a list of health conditions is weaved into the text after Synge mentions the health-loaded word "congestion." Firstly, he writes about "the tension of the mind" (209). Secondly, he links the calm following the storm to healing from fever as "[w]hen the sun rises there is a morning of almost supernatural radiance, and even the oldest men and women come out into the air with the joy of children who have recovered from a fever" (209). Thirdly, he explores the possible effect of the landscape on health: "This peculiar climate, acting on a population that is already lonely and dwindling, has caused or increased a tendency to nervous depression among the people, and every degree of sadness, from that of the man who is merely mournful to that of the man who has spent half his life in the madhouse, is common among these hills" (209). Fourthly, he records the words of an old man who "went on to tell me how different the country had been when he was a young man" and who says, "[N]ow all this country is gone lonesome and bewildered, and there's no man knows what ails it" (210). Fifthly, he adds that "[i]ntense nervousness is common also with much younger women" (211). The geography of "The Oppression of the Hills" is interesting. Despite Synge's fear that modernisation might create homogeneity, Synge's use of Hiberno-English itself homogenises English as spoken in Ireland at the turn of the century. That is, his "peasantry" (whether in Wicklow, Mayo, or Kerry) speak a "synthetic" dialect. He does the same with the geography of rural Ireland. His representation of Wicklow and its denizens is largely indistinguishable from that of the Congested Districts. Modernist "primitivism" runs the risk—that of reifying the other (the rural Irish, in this case) as "other" to metropolitan modernity, but, in so doing, losing that other's specificity. Synge believed that the west of Ireland would lose its power if it became like anywhere else and, evidently, for him, illness was an integral part of the rural identity that was bound up with the environment itself and elicited a certain type of power.

The "Congested" part of the "Congested Districts Board" did not only apply to the remote areas of Ireland but it also had personal and metaphorical associations for Synge in a medical sense. Alternatively, the medical definition of "congested" is to be "[o]vercharged with an unnatural accumulation of blood" and "affected with congestion," which is a complication that is often associated with the lungs and chest ("Congested"; *OED*). Lung congestion is a "distention of blood vessels in the lungs and filling of the alveoli with blood as a result of an infection, high blood pressure, or cardiac insufficiencies (*i.e.*, inability of the heart to function adequately)" ("Lung Congestion"; *Encyclopædia Britannica*). Due to his asthma and experience of chronic illness, Synge would have been aware of the medical denotation of the word "congested" and he would have been all too familiar with its physical sensation of suffocation, a feeling that did not fit with the rural Irish districts that had never been congested in the first place and did not require the "cure" of decongestion.

* * *

At the beginning of Synge's *The Well of the Saints*, his only play that pays substantial attention to illness and healing, the scene opens with a dialogue between the two blind characters. It becomes clear that these blind protagonists have a false mental image of themselves. They are blind to their own appearances as Mary Doul believes that she has "white beautiful skin" and Martin Doul contemplates, "[I]t'd be a grand thing if we could see ourselves for one hour, or a minute itself, the way we'd know surely we were the finest man, and the finest woman, of the seven counties of the east" (71, 73; act 1). Timmy, "a middle-aged, almost elderly, but vigorous smith," then enters the scene bearing the good news that a Saint is coming to heal their blindness (69; "Persons"). A "handsome girl" named Bride and Molly Byrne, a "fine-looking girl with fair hair," are entrusted to carry the cure (69; "Persons").[10] They are "*carrying water-can, Saint's bell, and cloak*" and Molly states that "I've holy water here from the grave of the four saints of the west, will have you cured in a short while and seeing like ourselves" (83; act 1). When the Saint arrives, he says to Martin Doul that "I'll cure you first, and then I'll come for your wife" and that "[w]e'll go up now into the church, for I must say a prayer to the Lord" (91; act 1). Meanwhile, Timmy "*anxiously*" reflects that "I'm thinking it was bad work we did when we let on she [Mary Doul] was fine-looking, and not a wrinkled wizened hag the way she is" (91, 93; act 1). When Martin Doul's sight is recovered, he declares that "I see now surely," but he "doesn't know her [his wife] at all"; and Mary Doul reacts in a similar way and an argument ensues (93, act 1). The blind protagonists' rejection of the cure is a comic twist that would cause audiences to reflect on what really is a boon and a blessing. In this play, Synge asks the question, how does one help people, and what counts as help? What is enacted and transacted among the characters on the stage has much wider ramifications.

Synge was highly sceptical about the Congested Districts Board that did not listen to people and imposed charity. In this light, it is worth returning to Synge's figure of the Saint in *The Well of the Saints*, whom the playwright engineers to restore the sight of the blind couple without

[10] Byrne is an Irish surname that is identified with County Wicklow.

stopping to think what will make them happy. With their restored sight, both Martin and Mary Doul return to work: "*Martin Doul is sitting near forge, cutting sticks*" and "*Mary Doul comes in unnoticed on right with a sack filled with green stuff on her arm*" (103, 107; act 2). Occupied with exterior appearance and dissatisfied with their everyday duties, the couple waste their gift of sight and eventually their eyes start "dimming again" (105; act 2). Timmy again communicates a solution as "[t]he saint's come to marry the two of us, and I'm after speaking a word for yourselves, the way he'll be curing you now, for if you're a foolish man itself, I do be pitying you, for I've a kind heart, when I think of you sitting dark again, and you after seeing a while, and working for your bread" (137; act 3). The Saint says, "It's many a time those that are cured with the well of the four beauties of God lose their sight when a time is gone, but those I cure a second time go on seeing till the hour of death" (139; act 3). He then "*takes the cover from his can*" and informs the couple that "I've a few drops only left of the water, but, with the help of God, it'll be enough for the two of you, and let you kneel down now upon the road" (139; act 3). It is not hard to see that Synge views the figure of the Saint as a beneficent authority doling out homogenising charity like the Congested Districts Board. In this way of understanding the play, in Synge's eyes, rebelliousness becomes a proof of life and individuality.

Martin Doul openly rejects the Saint's offer of healing and poses a rhetorical question: "Would you have her looking on me, and saying hard words to me, till the hour of death?" (143; act 3). Mary Doul tells the Saint to "[l]et us be as we are, holy father, and then we'll be known again as the people is happy and blind, and we'll be having an easy time with no trouble to live, and we getting half-pence on the road," but then Mat Simon, another character who is present, "*half persuaded*" her to accept the cure (143; act 3). When the Saint is in the process of curing Mary Doul's eyes, Martin Doul "*with a sudden movement strikes the can from [the] Saint's hand and sends it rocketing across stage*" (147; act 3). Martin Doul says, "I'm thinking it's a good right ourselves have to be sitting blind, hearing a soft wind turning round the little leaves of the spring and feeling the sun" (149; act 3). Martin and Mary Doul resolve to go "to the towns of the south" and then the play ends with the marriage of "Molly Byrne and Timmy the smith" (149; act 3). The ending of the play in a marriage enables a gauze-thin comic covering to be pulled over the play but, in the minds of audiences, the violent action of Martin Doul is the piece's true denouement.

At the resolution, there are two forms of union: one is healthy, and the other is unhealthy. Timmy and Molly Byrne look forward to a fruitful marriage, whereas Martin and Mary Doul await a life of exile due to their own poor choices. Mary Doul "*despondingly*" talks about her and Martin's new reality of "walking with a slough of wet on the one side and a slough of wet on the other, and you going a stony path with a north wind blowing behind" (149, 151; act 3). Timmy and Molly Byrne, however, "come up now into the church" and choose marriage (151; act 3). The secondary characters are getting married and this keeps the play within the genre. Timmy and the Saint are the final speakers:

> TIMMY. There's a power of deep rivers with floods in them where you do have to be lepping the stones and you going to the south, so I'm thinking the two of them will be drowned together in a short while, surely.
> SAINT. They have chosen their lot, and the Lord have mercy on their souls. [*He rings his bell*]. And let the two of you come up now into the church, Molly Byrne and Timmy the smith, till I make your marriage and put my blessing on you all. (151; act 3)

With this, the Saint attempts to re-establish the order for which he stands: health and piety, the whole and the holy. One relationship is likely to lead to death; the other relationship leads to life and continued life through children. Traditionally, comic plays end in marriage as a form of resolution, a tradition which goes back at least as far as Sophocles, and it is present in every Shakespeare comedy. As was the convention among Attic dramatists, Sophocles confined himself to tragedy and wrote no comedies (if one excludes the Satyr play *Ichneutae*, and this is not a comedy in the manner of Greek Old or New Comedy). The kind of harmonious "comic" conclusion that Synge overrides in his play dates from Menander and Greek New Comedy, an influence on Roman comic dramatists Plautus and Terence, and which percolates from hence to Renaissance comic drama. Synge's two-tiered ending, one of marriage and the other of self-exile, presents the audience with two versions of "sight" that they look upon with their own eyes. Comedy is the funny twin of Synge's subjective moralising because he used humour to reflect on how people can be helped and whether this can be achieved by giving the remote Irish people what they want rather than what approved authorities think they need. The play leaves it ambiguous as to which resolution Synge thought was right or preferable. He appears to overshadow the conventional comic ending of marriage and children. Synge's true comic ending seems bound up in Mary and Martin's free wanderings on the roads.[11]

This idea of ultimate happiness accords with Synge's own life. In the *Autobiography of J. M. Synge: Constructed from the Manuscripts* (written 1896–1898 and 1907; published 1965), later reprinted in his *Collected Works, Volume II: Prose* (1982), Synge writes about returning to school following an absence due to illness in his early years[12]:

> I was now at school again, but ill continually. This ill health led to a curious resolution which has explained in some measure all my subsequent evolution. Without knowing, or, as far as I can remember, hearing anything about doctrines of heredity I surmised that unhealthy parents should have unhealthy children—my rabbit breeding may have put the idea into my head. Therefore, I said, I am unhealthy, and if I marry I will have unhealthy children. But I will never create beings to suffer as I am suffering, so I will never marry. I do not know how old I was when I came to this decision, but I was between thirteen and fifteen and it caused me horrible misery. (*CW*2: 9)

He continues to write that "[t]he following spring I had measles and gave up school finally" and "[w]hen I recovered I began to collect moths and butterflies and other insects, a pursuit which kept me engrossed for several years" (*CW*2: 9). It is evident that illness was one of Synge's first comprehensive memories because he recalls, "My promotion to knickerbockers and a severe cough or croup came about the time that I began to remember coherently" (3). Ill health is the thread that weaves Synge's mindset together. Over time, he developed his own reaction to it because, in response to bouts of illness, he would either "wander about among the fields" or "collect moths and butterflies" (6, 9). Synge used his illness as a passport to an outside world, where he hid from responsibility. In his play, like Synge, Martin and Mary Doul are childless. Synge, who decided not to marry and have children due to fears of passing on his own ill health to them, perhaps believed that the blind couple's childlessness represented

[11] This is also the ending of *The Playboy of the Western World* (1907), which can be read in Synge's *Collected Works, Volume IV: Plays, Book II* (1968), edited by Ann Saddlemyer (173; act 3).

[12] In the introduction, editor Alan Price writes, "The material from which the *Autobiography* is constructed is taken from a note-book (No. 15) written between 1896 and 1898, sheets, (No. 21), written about 1898, and typewritten sheets of revisions, made probably in 1907, of a small part of the preceding material (No. 52)" (*Autobiography* 8).

freedom at the end of the play in contrast to the married couple Molly and Tim.

* * *

Like other writers, Synge responded to the Congested Districts Board with scepticism. In his book *J. M. Synge: Nature, Politics, Modernism*, Seán Hewitt argues that "[l]ike AE [born George William Russell], Synge was concerned that the CDB's [Congested Districts Board's] attempts to improve the material situation of the peasantry would lead to the destruction of their 'rich humanity'; unlike AE, Synge did not counter this by advocating the improvement of the peasantry on Christian and cooperative terms" (151; AE, "The best place for co-operation" qtd. in Hewitt 151). Hewitt writes, "For both men, self-help was the ultimate goal; however, where AE saw in the Congested Districts a place where 'the people are the most backward and most teachable,' Synge preferred to see the peasantry as recalcitrant, and as an opposition to the standardizing improvement schemes enacted under constructive unionist policy" (151; AE, "Local Organisation" qtd. in Hewitt 151). This can be seen in the contrast between AE's poem "The Well of All-Healing" (1897) and Synge's play *The Well of the Saints*.

In a version of AE's poem that was printed in 1897 in a periodical titled *A Celtic Christmas*, the first line reads, "There's a cure for all things in the well at Ballykeele."[13] In his later *Collected Poems* (1913), perhaps partly due to Yeats's revisions, this becomes, "There's a cure for sorrow in the well at Ballylee" (197). Synge believed that the Congested Districts Board's "methods of improvement are seen in terms contrary to local, natural processes" and that "[t]he force of unionism and joyless work leads the people to physical and mental degeneration" (Hewitt, 155, 157). Synge disliked the way that the Congested Districts Board treated the landscape and the people who live in it, forcing them to undertake unpleasant occupations like stone-breaking instead of performing traditional labour of the locality such as kelp-making.

Synge expresses his dissatisfaction with working life in *The Well of the Saints*, especially at the resolution when Martin Doul says, "We're going surely, for if it's a right some of you have to be working and sweating the

[13] See my own chapter, "Thoor Ballylee: Healing and Recovery," which contains a copy of this poem.

like of Timmy the smith, ... I'm thinking it's a good right ourselves have to be sitting blind" (149; act 3). As expressed in the essay "The Boat Builders" in *In Wicklow, West Kerry and Connemara*, Synge thought that "the people should be left as free as possible to arrange their houses and way of life as it pleases them" (*CW* 2: 315). In "Possible Remedies," the final essay in this posthumous collection, Synge suggests potential solutions and writes that "[i]t is not easy to improve the state of the people in the congested districts by any particular remedy or set of remedies" (*CW* 2: 339). Synge had intended collecting these pieces of travel writing in book form but died before doing so; Yeats was instrumental in collecting them as a "single" work. Hewitt notes, "Importantly, however, Synge advocates self-government as the measure preliminary to all others" (*Synge* 167). Synge took societal healing into his own hands and hoped that his idea for political selfhood could be a potential salve that he could apply to modernisation.

In *J. M. Synge and Travel Writing of the Irish Revival* (2017), Giulia Bruna argues that "[d]espite a nostalgia for a pre-colonial past, the Revival was thus a product of modernity and modernization" and "[f]ar from being only backward looking, Revival activists and movements embraced modernity and technological advancements for the benefit of their work of cultural recovery" (55). Synge's own modernity is evident in his photography and also in the fact that he was unusual (especially as a man) in using a typewriter at this date. His ethnography (as explored by Gregory Castle, among others), especially on the Aran Islands, is also a "modern" intervention into the traditional culture he seeks to document. Hewitt writes, "The focus on a 'natural link' between the people and the 'world that is about them' is a key concern throughout Synge's writings, and the disruption of this link through modernization becomes the fundamental basis for his opposition to systematic schemes of 'improvement'" (*Synge* 41; *CW* 2: 58–59, 93). For Synge, that is where the blindness is: improvement schemes that refuse to question actions or motives and impose a single centralised notion of what is right and beneficial.

Synge complicates matters and halts the recovery process using the patients' unappreciative reaction to health and wellness. Synge's focal point for the play is an authentic well that exists in Inishmore (Inis Mór), one of the Aran Islands that lies at the mouth of Galway Bay, which is a place that he frequented to collect folklore. By bringing this well to "[*s*]*ome lonely mountainous district in the east of Ireland, one or more centuries ago*," he relocates it to County Wicklow and thus "Aranises" the rest of Ireland from west to east and present to past (69; "Scene"). This re-inflects my point about "The Oppression of the Hills," which, although set in Wicklow, in its use of the word "congested" suggests the concerns of other travel journalism that Synge wrote about the "congested districts" properly defined. In doing this, he also brings the well to himself as his family resided in County Wicklow from the eighteenth century, which fits the time frame in which his play is set. Holy wells, which are widespread and powerful places of healing in Ireland, are a useful lens with which to view medicine in Synge's works.

Whilst navigating the east and west and a few past centuries, Synge also harkens back to early mythology. There are parallels between Synge's *The Well of the Saints* and Yeats's epic poem *The Wanderings of Oisin* (1889). On the surface, both have strong thematic parallels: the Saint is similar to St. Patrick; Oisin, the headstrong and impetuous hero, was possibly connected in Synge's mind to the blind protagonists. The blind couple's resolution "to be lepping the stones" is reminiscent of the resolution to Yeats's *The Wanderings of Oisin* (151; act 3). Similarly, Oisin says that "[w]e will tear out the flaming stones [of Hell]" at the end of the poem (*VP* book 3, line 209). Just as the blind protagonists are childless, so is Oisin "[w]ithout laughter, a show unto children, alone with remembrance and fear" (line 218). Hewitt argues that "Synge's *The Well of the Saints* is designed specifically as Ossianic, and thus draws not only on Synge's predilection for dialectical writing but also on the Revivalist concern to tie the modern movement to a definably native tradition" (*Synge* 124). However, St. Patrick and Oisin are different to the Saint and the blind couple. St. Patrick tries to save the impulsive Oisin using words; the Saint attempts to permanently cure the reluctant blind couple using healing water.

Unlike the blind protagonists, Oisin laments the vulnerable condition of being "shaken with coughing and broken with old age and pain" (*VP* book 3, line 217). St. Patrick describes Oisin as being "bent, and bald, and blind" at the outset of the poem, and Oisin later portrays himself as being "weak and poor and blind" (book 1, line 1; book 2, line 203). Oisin recalls a time when he had some level of sight when he claims that "[i]t were sad to gaze on the blessèd and no man I loved of old there" because he missed the presence of the Fenians in Ireland (book 3, line 221). He does not rely on an ailment like blindness to go where he wants to be; rather, he uses the health that he has left to "go to Caoilte, and Conan, and Bran, Sceolan, Lomair, / And dwell in the house of the Fenians, be they in flames or at feast" (lines 223–24). On the other hand, Synge holds up his own version of hero in dialectic and he employs illness as a strange superpower that the blind couple use to become invisible to society and camouflage back into the landscape. Synge laces his play with ancient Irish mythology but, unlike Yeats, he provides two resolutions of differing health statuses for the audience to ponder. Synge highlights character and necessity of the ill, wounded, stubborn, and inassimilable.

Even though Synge's writing is ironic, he mentions very real places of healing. For example, in *The Well of the Saints*, the Saint asks Martin Doul a question: "Did you never set eyes on the summer and the fine spring in the places where the holy men of Ireland have built up churches to the Lord, ...?" (141; act 3). In response, in the 1905 edition of the play, Martin Doul replies, "Is it talking now you are of Knock and Ballavore?" (140; act 3).[14] In Knock, there was a Eucharistic and Marian Apparition, which caused healings that continue today. In *Knock: The Virgin's Apparition in Nineteenth-Century Ireland* (2008), Eugene Hynes writes that "[o]n August 21 1879, in a poor rural village in the western county of Mayo, over a dozen people saw a bright silvery-white light outside the gable of the local Catholic church and within the light the Virgin Mary, St. Joseph and a third figure they identified as St. John the Evangelist" (xiii). There was also the Risen Lamb that stood upon an altar in front of a cross. Hynes notes that "[a]ngels' wings surrounded the altar" (xiii). Liam úa Cadhain writes that "claims of cures were being constantly made by pilgrims who visited Knock after the report ... of the Apparition" (*Venerable Archdeacon Cavanagh* 92).[15] Marion Carroll, who had multiple sclerosis, was cured at Knock Shrine in 1989 and this healing was officially verified in 2019.[16] It is possible that Synge knew about the healings at Knock that occurred in his lifetime, as they were well reported, and this is perhaps why he mentions Knock in his play.

Traditional healing practices are at the heart of Synge's first three-act play *The Well of the Saints* (1905), as a character named the Saint travels Ireland with its healing waters. However, the waters' curative powers are not universally welcomed because the play's protagonists, Martin and

[14] In a footnote, editor Ann Saddlemyer notes that this line was deleted in future drafts (*CW* 2: 140; act 3).

[15] Venerable Archdeacon Cavanagh wrote a *Diary of Cures*, which he began on 31 October 1879. This manuscript, alongside letters that people sent to him describing cures that had happened to themselves or others, can be viewed in Knock Museum at Knock Shrine.

[16] See Marion Carroll and John Scally's *My Miracle Cure: An Extraordinary Story of Hope, Healing and the Power of Faith* (2020).

Mary Doul, ultimately reject the gift of sight. Though this seems inexplicable, Synge's ideas regarding the nature of modernity and development dovetail with this outcome. He ironically and irreverently uses the character of the Saint to represent the charitable impulse that might provide people with what they need—sight—but not what they want. Synge employs "sight" as a concept that distinguishes eyesight from mindsight, objective from subjective perspectives, and confirms his view of well-being as separate from good physical health.

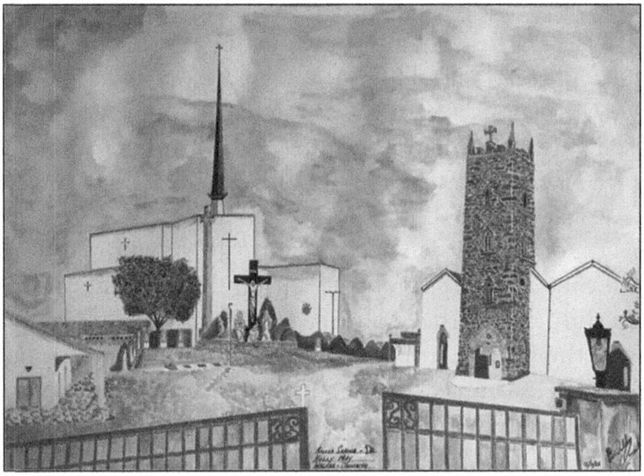

Knock Shrine

CHAPTER 7

Healing Wells in the Work of John Millington Synge

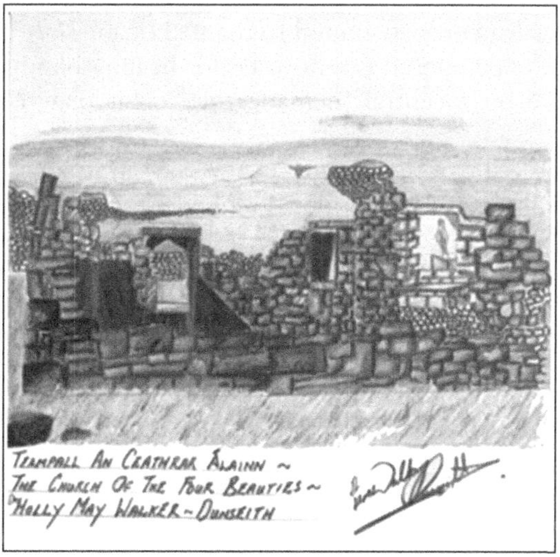

Teampall an Ceathrar Álainn—The Church of the Four Beauties

H. M. Walker-Dunseith, *Traditional Medicine in the Irish Literary Revival*, New Directions in Irish and Irish American Literature,
https://doi.org/10.1007/978-3-031-82459-3_7

John Millington Synge first visited the Well of the Four Beauties (Tobar an Ceathrar Álainn) on Inishmore (Inis Mór) in 1898, a place which was to become an inspiration for his play *The Well of the Saints* (1905). This well, dug into a field, encircled with stones, is in the middle of Inishmore, close to Corrúch village. It lies immediately to the south of the Church of the Four Beauties (Teampall an Ceathrar Álainn), where Saints Fursey, Brendan of Birr, Conall, and Berchán are reputedly buried. This site is alive with accounts of healing: the stone flags of the saints' graves themselves are said to have curative properties. According to his report of his visit in *The Aran Islands* (1906), before getting to this location, Synge "rested near the ruins of a house" and went "some distance to the north to visit one of the ancient beehive dwellings that is still in perfect preservation" (*CW* 2: 54).[1] Healing wells are prevalent in Ireland and there are many accounts of people being cured using the water from these wells.[2] Whilst some have reputations for remedying a variety of illnesses, others have more specialist cures attributed to them (Logan, *Holy Wells* 69). The well that Synge encountered is renowned for healing blindness, a malady that would take on a central thematic role in his play *The Well of the Saints* (1905).

Blindness has a literal significance in the play: in it, a character named the Saint goes about Ireland curing the blind. It also has a metaphorical importance: this play explores tropes of illumination and benightedness that were current during the Revival period, with its investment in national

[1] Synge may be referring to a dilapidated house in Killeaney, and the beehive dwelling was likely to have been the stone-built Clochan na Carraige that is situated in the middle of Kilmurvey and Onaght in Inishmore.

[2] For information about curing wells, see Patrick Logan's *The Holy Wells of Ireland* (1980), the *National Folklore Collection* (*NFC*), and *The Schools' Manuscript Collection* (*NFCS*). For example: in the latter collection, County Mayo informant Kate Hastings states that "[t]here is a well in Knock and in Kilgeever where people are cured from certain ailments," which includes "[p]eople that are dumb, deaf, blind, cripples and people with sores" ("Ailments" 36; *NFCS* 0138D: 34–37; Kate Hastings, Leenavesta, County Mayo. Collector: Caitlín Ní Oistín, St. Bridget's (school), Derrymore, County Mayo, 5 April 1938. Teacher: Máire Uí hOistín). The "well in Knock" that Hastings refers to is most likely St. Patrick's Well (Tobar Phádraig) in Carrownedan in Aghamore near Knock. In reference to this same well, Paddy O'Brien informs that "[i]t is said that people ha[ve] been cured of eye trouble from bat[h]ing [sic] in the water" ("St. Patrick's Well" 251; *NFCS* 0107: 250–252; Collector's father, parent, Holywell Lower, Ballyhaunis, County Mayo. Collector: Paddy O'Brien, Scoil Mhuire, Béal Átha hAmhnais (school), Ballyhaunis, County Mayo, c. 1937–1939. Teacher: S. T. Ó Maolagáin).

narratives of redemptive epochal change. Synge's own imagination presents challenges to received narratives of the Revival period: he is primarily an explorer of paradoxically opposed states rather than a teller of heroic tales. And so, in Synge's play, the desirability of illumination in darkness itself is thrown into question. The two chief protagonists of *The Well of the Saints*, the blind Martin and Mary Doul, would rather be blind than face the world around them: "For it's a raw, beastly day we do have each day, till I do be thinking it's *well* for the blind don't be seeing the like of them grey clouds driving on the hill, and don't be looking on people with their noses red, the like of your nose, and their eyes weeping, and watering, the like of your eyes, God help you, Timmy the smith" (*CW* 3: 105; act 2; emphasis added). Synge's characters are not concerned with the ability to *see*, because they are more preoccupied with the desire to *unsee* the modern world. Blindness might, in spite of everything, be a blessed state.

Though the lives and landscapes that inspired Synge make his work in some ways paradigmatic of Revivalist practice, there is a complication at the heart of his writing. In the worlds of Synge's plays, opposites and irony are given free rein, and this makes them a rich and challenging resource for those who are curious about the Irish Revival. The distance between a prose passage Synge wrote about an occasion of miraculous healing by Aran well-water, and the obdurate Martin and Mary Doul's resistance to being healed by the same substance, is informative about the fractures and complications that were present both in Synge's own imagination, and in Ireland at the turn of the twentieth century.

In *The Aran Islands*, an assemblage of journal accounts focused on Synge's visits to the islands, the reader is presented with a benign, even heart-warming, story of miraculous healing from a well.[3] In this account, Synge writes about an elderly blind man that he calls "old Mourteen" who shows him around the area (*CW* 2: 54). Synge writes, "In spite of the charm of my teacher, the old blind man I met the day of my arrival, I have decided to move on to Inishmaan, where Gaelic is more generally used, and the life is perhaps the most primitive that is left in Europe" (53). He remembers that "I spent all this last day with my blind guide, looking at

[3] Readers cannot always trust Synge's supposedly factual prose accounts, as Seán Hewitt notices in his book *J. M. Synge: Nature, Politics, Modernism* (2021), when he writes about how Synge sees a bird and a golf ball (137). Hewitt applies a caveat that reads: "It is unlikely that either of the two incidents [pertaining to the bird and the golf ball] are true to life, since both were first written down by Synge years after his final trip to the Aran Islands and seem to have been prompted by his researches in the Congested Districts" (137).

the antiquities that abound in the west or north-west of the island" (54). The blind man took him to the well at Inishmore, where another old man came and imparted knowledge that would influence Synge's future play written seven years later. He writes an entry about this moment that struck him on his very first trip there in 1898:

> A couple of miles from this village [an unnamed village that contained a "slated house"] we turned aside to look at an old ruined church of the Ceathair Aluinn (The Four Beautiful Persons), and a holy well near it that is famous for cures of blindness and epilepsy.
>
> As we sat near the well a very old man came up from a cottage near the road, and told me how it had become famous.
>
> "A woman of Sligo had a son who was born blind, and one night she dreamed that she saw an island with a blessed well in it that could cure her son. She told her dream in the morning, and an old man said it was of Aran she was after dreaming.
>
> "She brought her son down by the coast of Galway, and came out in a curagh, and landed below where you see a bit of a cove.
>
> "She walked up then to the house of my father—God rest his soul—and she told them what she was looking for.
>
> "My father said that there was a well like what she had dreamed of, and that he would send a boy along with her to show her the way.
>
> "'There's no need, at all,' said she; 'haven't I seen it all in my dream?'"
>
> "Then she went out with the child and walked up to this well, and she kneeled down and began saying her prayers. Then she put her hand out for the water, and put it on his eyes, and the moment it touched him he called out: 'O mother, look at the pretty flowers!'" (56–57)

Although this tale has a simple beauty to it, a note of uneasiness is perhaps made present by the fact that Synge's guide, "Old Mourteen," was himself still blind in spite of the presence of this miraculous water. The healing may not have worked for Mourteen or, like the blind couple in *The Well of the Saints*, he could have rejected the cure altogether. It is possible that this irony, unremarked on in the prose work, germinated in Synge's sardonic dramatic imagination. Whereas, in the story in *The Aran Islands*, as in received wisdom, the restoration of sight is longed-for and a cause of rejoicing, Synge's play is interested in the alluring capacities of darkness.

The origins of Synge's play go deeper, of course, than a single encounter in the Aran Islands. Synge's fascination with healing wells, and the transformative possibilities that they represent, perhaps stems from his own ailments that he experienced from childhood. According to Declan Kiberd, writing an account of Synge's life for the *Dictionary of Irish Biography* (2009), illness was a significant part of Synge's life:

> J. M. Synge was a frail child, constantly prone to sickness; and he resolved at an early age never to have children of his own, lest they inherit his maladies. Nonetheless, he was a lover of nature and the outdoors, becoming an active member of the Dublin Naturalists' Field Club (1886–8). He was educated mainly at home by a tutor, but at the age of 10 was sent to Mr Harrick's classical and English school, Upper Leeson St., Dublin. Ill health greatly affected his attendance and he was withdrawn after three years. He spent most summers on extended family holidays at Greystones, but was never allowed to swim, because of respiratory problems. (Kiberd, *DIB*)[4]

In his essay "J. M. Synge and the Ireland of his Time," written in September 1910, Yeats writes that "[w]hat blindness did for Homer, lameness for Hephaestus, asceticism for any saint you will, bad health did for him by making him ask no more of life than that it should keep him living, and above all perhaps by concentrating his imagination upon one thought, health itself" (*Essays and Introductions* 321). Yeats continues with an explanation of Synge's power that is similar to his one of Keats's: "I am certain that my friend's noble art, so full of passion and heroic beauty, is the victory of a man who in poverty and sickness created from the delight of expression, and in the contemplation that is born of the minute and delicate arrangement of images, happiness and health of mind" (321).[5] Synge becomes yet another figure in whom Yeats can find confirmation of his theory of the "anti-self"; he functions in Yeats's imagination much like Keats in "Ego Dominus Tuus" (1918). To Yeats, whose imagination was drawn to antimonies and contrasts long before he codified his preoccupations in the grand scheme of *A Vision* (1925), Synge's lack of health was

[4] Also, see W. J. McCormack's biography of Synge titled *Fool of the Family: A Life of J. M. Synge* (2000), which documents Synge's illness throughout his life. McCormack records Synge's retreats, for example: "Recovering from the mental stress of *The Playboy* riots yet also slipping into terminal illness, Synge tried Kerry again as a retreat in October 1907, but stayed only four days, assailed by asthma" (222).

[5] In "Ego Dominus Tuus" (1918), a dialogue poem about contrasting artists, Yeats writes, "What portion in the world can the artist have / Who has awakened from the common dream / But dissipation and despair? / And yet / No one denies to Keats love of the world; / Remember his deliberate happiness" (*VP* lines 49–53).

the wellspring of a paradoxical robustness in his imagination. In Synge's sickness, there was strength.

Synge, who had asthma, was familiar with illness; his health difficulties were subsequently woven into the fabric of his plays. In his autobiography, Synge remembers his early experience with ill health when he was approximately ten years old: "I was now going to school, but I had many holidays from ill health—six months about this time especially which were recommended on account of continual head-aches that I suffered from which gave us [Synge and his friend] a great deal of time to wander about among the fields near our houses" (*CW* 2: 6).[6] He claims, "We were left in complete liberty and never abused it" (6). The consonances between his own life and those of the blind protagonists of his plays are intriguing. Illness is liberation: in *The Well of the Saints*, Martin and Mary Doul are "happy and blind" and believe that "it's best we are this way, and we're not asking to see" (*CW* 3: 143, 139; act 3). Illness and the ability to abscond from the usages of the world—from what was nominally profitable or useful—and into nature, are connected in Synge's mind. There is something counterintuitive at work here: illness is not just an affliction to be borne. Synge speaks as if illness gave him the opportunity to immerse himself in nature, and he is willing to see possibilities in the anti-revival of his health.

* * *

In *The Well of the Saints*, Synge was using the Irish Literary Revival and the Abbey to question ideas that went to the heart of the Revival. One of these ideas is that the west was the home of a culture whose uncorrupted way of life could be redemptive of the more industrialised east and, at this date, not just the metropolitan east, but the even more industrialised north (Belfast). In her book *J. M. Synge and Travel Writing of the Irish Revival* (2017), Giulia Bruna writes that "the rural and most westward spots in the West of Ireland, where Irish was still more widely spoken, became a pilgrimage site for Revival artists and activists" (6). Declan Kiberd and P. J. Mathews, in *Handbook of the Irish Revival* (2016), aver that "[m]uch

[6] Synge is referring to "a friendship with a girl of my own age who was our neighbour" (*Autobiography* 17). In the 1965 edition of his autobiography, the sentence reads: "I was now going to school, but I had many holidays from ill-health—six months especially which were recommended on account of continual head-aches—that gave us scope to wander about among the fields near our houses" (17).

of the literature of the period is heavily invested in representing Ireland as a place of unsurpassed beauty and vitality—especially those regions on the western seaboard that were most affected by the Famine" (183).[7] The cultural dynamics of Ireland's geographies of east and west are a significant element of *The Well of the Saints*.

The Well of the Saints is not set in the storied west, but in Synge's ancestral county, Wicklow. Mary Doul refers to "the seven counties of the east," speaking of the counties that border the Irish Sea, stretching from Antrim and Down in the north, through Dublin and down to Wexford (129; act 3).[8] The phrase is a reminder that the play is set in Wicklow, which was not heavily populated at that time. Its mining industry (lead) was very far from developed; it had been stronger in the eighteenth century. Synge's essay, "A Landlord's Garden in County Wicklow," represents a picture of a decayed landlord class in a largely rural economy (*CW* 2: 230–33). The west of Ireland was a source of renewal. McCormack talks about Synge's essays on Wicklow constituting a "psychopathology" of the county, which would suggest the need for a "revival" from the west that the (eastern seaboard) old, blind couple reject (*Fool of the Family* 219). Molly, who is "*carrying* [*the*] *water-can*," says that "I've holy water here from the grave of the four saints of the west, will have you cured in a short while and seeing like ourselves—" (83; act 1). The water from the well is from the west: it is, according to ideas that were popular in Irish culture, including among his fellow artists, at the time Synge was writing, from a place of healing and Revival. However, Synge implies that there is something uncomfortable about this watery cure-all: Molly's promise to the blind Douls that they will soon be "seeing like ourselves" seems more like a threat of assimilation into collective blandness than the promise of a longed-for cure. It is of a piece of Synge's critique of the ideology of (aspects of) Revivalism that would prompt *The Playboy of the Western World* (1907), and account for the harsh reception of that play's depiction of the west by former Dáil Éireann president and writer Arthur Joseph Griffith (1871–1922) and his fellow nationalists.

[7] Blindness itself is a secondary illness of hunger and starvation; it is a famine-related illness and a complication caused by being deprived of food.

[8] There are now eight counties that form "[t]he East Coast & Midlands Region" and these are: "Kildare, Laois, Longford, Louth, Offaly, Meath, Westmeath and Wicklow" ("Regions of Ireland"; *Discovering Ireland*).

In the first act, Synge establishes the well as having western Irish associations, but then makes it clear that he relocates it to the east in his play, which is part of Synge's attempt to demystify this veneration of "the west" as a kind of idealised Revival-era *locus amoenus* or "pleasant place." Timmy initiates the conversation about the holy well:

> TIMMY. Did ever you hear tell of a place across a bit of the sea, where there is an island, and the grave of the four beautiful saints?
> MARY DOUL. I've heard people have walked round from the west and they speaking of that.
> TIMMY. [*impressively.*] There's a green ferny well, I'm told, behind of that place, and if you put a drop of the water out of it, on the eyes of a blind man, you'll make him see as *well* as any person is walking the world. (79; act 1; emphasis added)

Timmy is referring to Inishmore, the largest of the Aran Islands, where the Church of the Four Beauties is located. The "green ferny well," which is famed for curing blindness, is indeed "behind of that place," that is, south of the saints' burial place near where the fifteenth-century church remains standing. The idea that a western cure might save the eyes of the benighted east touches on some of the most treasured precepts of the Revival.

This is a complex issue, however, because Martin Doul rejects the water from the well that is offered for his healing. In Act One, the Saint cures the blind couple in the church. The Saint says that "with the power of the water I'm after bringing in a little curagh into Cashla Bay, [H]e'll have pity on you, and put sight into your eyes" and "[w]e'll go up now into the church, for I must say a prayer to the Lord" (91; act 1). At the resolution, the Saint offers the blind couple a second and permanent cure for their eyesight as "[i]t's many a time those that are cured with the well of the four beauties of God lose their sight when a time is gone, but those I cure a second time go on seeing till the hour of death" and "I've a few drops only left of the water, but, with the help of God, it'll be enough for the two of you, and let you kneel down now upon the road" (139; act 3). This time, the Saint says that "[y]ou can kneel down here, I'm saying, we'll not trouble this time going to the church" and "[k]neel down, I'm saying, the ground's dry at your feet" (139; act 3). The Saint speaks the healing blessing: "With the power of the water from the grave of the four beauties of God, with the power of this water, I'm saying, that I put upon your eyes——" (147; act 3). However, in the middle of the cure, Martin Doul, sinfully, "*with a sudden movement strikes the can from* [*the*] *Saint's hand and sends it rocketing across stage*" and he "heard the little splash of the water you [the Saint] had there in the can" (147, 149; act 3). The dry road on which they kneel, rather than the blind couple themselves, receive the blessing.

Was Synge dramatising a repudiation of the lore, language, practices, and stories that he himself had returned with from the west? We know Synge was interested in healing lore from the Atlantic seaboard. The Saint goes to the Well of the Four Beauties to bring healing water to the east, Synge goes to the west to take ideas and culture to the east, and the Abbey Theatre brings Revival to the east of Ireland. Synge mentions a traditional cure in his collection of essays called *In Wicklow, West Kerry and Connemara* (1911).[9] In his chapter "In West Kerry," Synge records a conversation with a fisherman named Maurice. He recalls, "We began to talk of fevers and sicknesses and doctors—these little villages are often infested with typhus—and Maurice spoke about the traditional cures" (*CW* 2: 246). Maurice specifies a particular cure that Synge describes:

> "There is a plant," he said, "which is the richest that is growing out of the ground, and in the old times the women used to be giving it to their children till they'd be growing up seven feet maybe in height. Then the priests and doctors began taking everything to themselves and destroyed the old knowledge, and that is a poor thing; for you know *well* it was the Holy Mother of God who cured her own Son with plants the like of that, and said after that no mother should be without a plant for ever to cure her child. Then she threw out the seeds of it over the whole world, so that it's growing every place from that day to this." (246; emphasis added)

Being closely acquainted with illness himself, this conversation was likely to have appealed to Synge, who had suffered from weak health since childhood. There are Revival-era echoes in the old man's speech as Revival writers seemed to believe that the religiosity and science of a newer era had destroyed what was salutary about the past and that the west of Ireland could be restorative of older and better practices that had been buried beneath what Yeats called, in his poem "The Statues" (1938), the "filthy modern tide" (*VP* line 29). The west of Ireland contained knowledge, practices, and beliefs that were restorative to what was, in the eyes of

[9] This title is significant as it conjoins his native eastern Wicklow with two locations from the west.

Revival-era writers, a fallen modern world. But the rejection of the cure by the Douls suggests that Synge's approach to the west was not as simple as this narrative of a holy west and a fallen east would suggest.

* * *

Yeats and Synge are not the only Revival-era writers who are interested in healing wells. In Jane Lady Wilde's short story "The Horned Women," which is placed in her collection *Ancient Legends, Mystic Charms, and Superstitions of Ireland* (1887) and is retold in Yeats's *Fairy and Folk Tales of the Irish Peasantry* (1888), a well has supernatural protective qualities. In Yeats's version of this narrative, which is essentially the same as Wilde's except for a few grammatical changes, a group of witches impose upon the house of "[a] RICH woman" and ask her to "make us a cake" (165, 166). The woman "searched for a vessel to bring water from the well that she might mix the meal and make the cake, but she could find none" so "she took the sieve and went to the well; but the water poured from it, and she could fetch none for the cake, and she sat down by the well and wept" (166). Rescuing her, it is "the Spirit of the Well" that is the "voice" that speaks to the woman and gives her instructions as to how to get the witches to leave the house and "bade the mistress of the house to enter and prepare her home against the enchantments of the witches if they returned again" (167). Wilde's story is a familiar tale of a well that is salutary, enabling an afflicted person to lift a curse.

Augusta Gregory, too, draws from the rich history of wells as sources of curing in Irish life. In her introduction to *The Kiltartan Poetry Book: Prose Translations from the Irish* (1919), Gregory writes:

> Even my own home "sweet Coole demesne" has been transfigured in songs of the neighbourhood; and a while ago an old woman asking alms at the door while speaking of a monastery near Athenry broke into a chant of praise that has in it perhaps some memory of the Well of Healing at the world's end that helped the gods to new strength in their great battle at Moytura. "Three barrels there are with water, and to see the first barrel boiling it is certain you will get a cure. Water there does be rushing down; you to stop you could hear it talking; to go there you would get cured of anything unless it might be the stroke of the Fool." (16)

Gregory is referring to a specific story in ancient Irish mythology. *Cath Maige Tuired: The Second Battle of Mag Tuired* is a manuscript that Gerard Murphy identifies as "the product of an eleventh or twelfth-century redactor working mainly upon ninth-century material" ("Notes on *Cath Maige Tuired*" 195). This manuscript is a two-tiered narrative about a primary battle between the Tuatha Dé Danann and the Fomorians and a secondary battle that happened in the past when the former victoried over the Fir Bolgs and acquired Irish kingship. In this story, one of the medicinal focal points is a healing well that restores and revives the warriors. The physicians "cast their mortally-wounded men into it as they were struck down; and they were alive when they came out" (*Cath Maige Tuired* 55). As "every man put a stone into the well," this is the "reason the cairn is called Ochtríallach's Cairn" yet "another name for that well is Loch Luibe, because Dían Cécht put into it every herb that grew in Ireland" (57). In *A Book of Saints and Wonders* (1907), Gregory frequently mentions healing wells, some of which cure eyesight such as St. Brigit's well at Liscannor in County Clare.[10] In "Book Three: Blessed Patrick of the Bells," Gregory writes a story about "the [Hidden] Well of Usnach that was called the Whitebrimmed" that was inhabited by "eight beautiful speckled salmon" (67). It is possible that this mythological Fenian narrative inspired Gregory's children's play *The Golden Apple* (1916) in so far as the King of Spain's daughter's "five brothers ... are turned to fishes in the well," specifically trout (*Selected Plays* 245; act 2, sc. 1). In "Book Five: Great Wonders of the Olden Time," in a story titled "The Birth of Colman of Aidhne," Gregory records a healing well in Kiltartan that cures blindness and lameness (*Saints and Wonders* 169–70). Wells and healing and blindness are linked in the Revival-era mind.

* * *

Yeats's later play *The Cat and the Moon*, written a decade after Synge's death, clearly owes much to the work of his friend. Yeats's play was written

[10] In "Book One: Brigit, The Mary of the Gael," in a subsection titled "She Remembers the Poor," Gregory describes "St. Brigit's well" at Liscannor in County Clare that cures the eyes amongst other illnesses (13–15). Gregory writes, "But if Brigit belonged to the east, it is not in the west she is forgotten, and the people of Burren and of Corcomruadh and Kinvara go every year to her blessed well that is near the sea, praying and remembering her" (13). She adds, "And in that well there is a little fish that is seen every seven years, and whoever sees that fish is cured of every disease" (13).

in 1917, published in 1924, and first performed in 1931. Yeats's play, like Synge's, includes a well, or rather "*a patterned curtain suggesting Saint Colman's Well*" (*VPl* 792). The play features a Blind Beggar and a Lame Beggar that meet a saint (referred to as a Holy Man) who offers to heal them (*VPl* 792). The Blind Beggar decides to "be cured of my blindness," but the Lame Beggar resolves to "stay lame" and "be blessed" (lines 156, 188–89).

Addressing the beggars, the First Musician asks, "Will you be cured or will you be blessed?" (lines 153–54). When the Lame Beggar in *The Cat and the Moon* decides that "I will stay lame" and "I will be blessed," this echoes Martin Doul's decision to keep his disability (lines 188–89). The Blind Beggar's choice to "be cured of my blindness" parallels Mary Doul, who is perhaps partially willing for her sight to be healed in Synge's play (line 156). The Blind Beggar observes that "[t]here is many gives money to a blind man" and, similarly, Martin Doul concludes that he was given more money for his blindness than for his work (lines 54–55). At the end of Synge's *The Well of the Saints*, the Saint's blessing is bestowed on the road instead of the Irish couple as the holy water is spilled. In Yeats's *The Cat and the Moon*, the First Musician tells the Lame Beggar, who chooses to "be blessed" instead of "be cured," that he "must bless the road" (line 275). However, the parallels between these plays go beyond accompanying elements. Questions of the benefits of both healing and sickness are central to both Synge's and Yeats's plays.

* * *

Both Synge's *The Well of the Saints* and Yeats's *At the Hawk's Well* (1917) share cohering images and both writers utilise healing wells in different ways; there is a differing significance of the well to each Irish Revival writer. Yeats's one-act play focuses on rejuvenation and the search for a curing water that fills the well at certain intervals in time. At the exposition, a first musician speaks about "[t]he withered leaves of the hazel" that "[h]alf choke the dry bed of the well" and describes "[t]he guardian of the well" who is "[w]orn out from raking its dry bed" and "[w]orn out from gathering up the leaves" (*VPl* lines 23–25, 27–28). The musician then concentrates on a different character and says, "That old man climbs up hither, / Who has been watching by his well / These fifty years. / He is all doubled up with age" (lines 39–42). Cuchulain, who is "Sualtim's son" and a young man, then appears and speaks about water from a well that the old man has been trying to find for fifty years (line 84).

Yeats, when he represented himself through his proxy Cuchulain, tended to see his life as one of heroic struggle. When he wrote *At the Hawk's Well*, he is turning his back on the naturalism of the "peasant plays" of the Abbey, and he is seeking—through his immersion in the Japanese Noh drama that Ezra Pound had from 1912 introduced him to—an "elitist" avant-garde drama to oppose the dominant dramatic realism of this period. Yeats's essay "A People's Theatre: A Letter to Lady Gregory" (1919) in *The Irish Dramatic Movement* (1899–1919) reveals "certain thoughts that have made me believe that the Abbey Theatre can never do all we had hoped" (*CW* 8: 124). He writes that "[w]e set out to make a 'People's Theatre,' and in that we have succeeded" yet "I did not know until very lately that there are certain things, dear to both our hearts, which no 'People's Theatre' can accomplish" (124). Yeats decides, "As a drawing is defined by its outline and taste by its rejections, I too must reject and draw an outline about the thing I seek; and say that I seek, not a theatre but the theatre's anti-self, an art that can appease all within us that becomes uneasy as the curtain falls and the house breaks into applause" (133). He states that "I want to create for myself an unpopular theatre and an audience like a secret society where admission is by favour and never to many" and "I desire a mysterious art, always reminding and half-reminding those who understand it of dearly loved things, doing its work by suggestion, not by direct statement, a complexity of rhythm, colour, gesture, not space-pervading like the intellect but a memory and a prophecy" (131–32). Thus, he turned *At the Hawk's Well* into a little theatre production with a cultivated audience in an aristocratic house in London. In his notes to the play, Russell K. Alspach confirms that "'At the Hawk's Well' was performed for the first time in April, 1916, in a friend's drawing-room, and only those who cared for poetry were invited" and "[a] few days later it was revived in Lady Islington's big drawing-room at Chesterfield Gardens for the benefit of a war charity" (*VPl* 416). There is a dialogue between the young and old man, and Cuchulain asks the elderly character to take him to the healing well:

> Lead me to what I seek, a well wherein
> Three hazels drop their nuts and withered leaves,
> And where a solitary girl keeps watch
> Among grey boulders. He who drinks, they say,
> Of that miraculous water lives for ever. (lines 98–102)

However, the old man replies that "I have lain in wait / For more than fifty years, to find it empty, / Or but to find the stupid wind of the sea / Drive round the perishable leaves" (lines 112–15). The young man understands that "[s]o it seems / There is some moment when the water fills it" (line 115–16). The old man, too, sought after the well when he was "young in body and in mind" and he recalls that "I waited the miraculous flood, I waited / While the years passed and withered me away" (lines 129, 132–33). His memories carry the bleak overtones of the Irish Famine as "I have snared the birds for food and eaten grass / And drunk the rain, and neither in dark nor shine / Wandered too far away to have heard the plash" (lines 134–36). The "*Guardian of the Well*" is a "Woman of the Sidhe" who prevents them from attaining their goal (lines 146, 161). As "*the Guardian of the Well has begun to dance, moving like a hawk*," this causes both men to fall asleep and the musicians sing that "[h]e has lost what may not be found / Till men heap his burial-mound / And all the history ends" (lines 212, 224–26). The continued lamenting musical tones echo the life that the blind couple could have lived in Synge's *The Well of the Saints*: "He might have lived at his ease, / An old dog's head on his knees, / Among his children and friends" (lines 227–29). This chorus, sung by the Musicians, consider if the characters would have been happier if they had not searched for the water.

In Synge's play, which similarly has a shared theme of futility, the Douls do not want the cure. It is interesting that Yeats's Cuchulain ends up not drinking from the well for very different reasons from the Douls. Both Yeats and Synge start from this point. Two elements are being questioned in the rejection of the well's water: Synge experiments with the possibility of whether people can be made to improve despite their own capacities and abilities, and he questions the Revival itself. In *In Wicklow, West Kerry and Connemara* (1911), he writes that "[o]ne feels then, perhaps a little later, that it is part of the misfortune of Ireland that nearly all the characteristics which give colour and attractiveness to Irish life are bound up with a social condition that is near to penury" (*CW* 2: 286). Referring to this line in *J. M. Synge: Nature, Politics, Modernism* (2021), Seán Hewitt comments, "[I]t is clear that the threat of standardization implicit in 'improvement' schemes is seen by him as a threat to both aesthetics and artistic potential" (155). The characters in *At the Hawk's Well* think that the well will lift a curse, but they conclude that the search for the cure is the curse as the Old Man tells the "[a]ccursed dancers," who prevent them from reaching the well, that "you have stolen my life" (line 234). Yeats implies that the search itself has cursed the characters. This play is an exploration of the costs of heroic action, and the disturbing possibility of its futility. For Yeats's protagonist, as for Synge's Douls, the desirability of the well's water is the occasion for significant doubt in the minds of the audience.

The roots of this play go back a long way. Yeats's first popular success as a poet, "The Lake Isle of Innisfree," is a story that itself concerns bubbling water in the west of Ireland. In "Book I: Four Years: 1887-1891" (1921) within his autobiography *The Trembling of the Veil* (1922), Yeats writes an account of his encounter with water in London that, although in a very different place, nonetheless reminded him of the gushing waters in his home in Sligo:

> Sometimes I told myself very adventurous love-stories with myself for hero, and at other times I planned out a life of lonely austerity, and at other times mixed the ideals and planned a life of lonely austerity mitigated by periodical lapses. I had still the ambition, formed in Sligo in my teens, of living in imitation of [Henry David] Thoreau on Innisfree, a little island in Lough Gill, and when walking through Fleet Street very homesick I heard a little tinkle of water and saw a fountain in a shop-window which balanced a little ball upon its jet, and began to remember lake water. From the sudden remembrance came my poem "Innisfree," my first lyric with anything in its rhythm of my own music. (*Autobiographies* 139)

Somehow, mysteriously, Yeats is aligning his first success as a poet with an image of rising water, and with the west of Ireland. It is intriguing that it is in London—*the* urban megalopolis at this date—that Yeats is (via what is a cheap advertising gimmick in a shopfront window) drawn to the rejuvenating potential of Sligo (and thus the west); Yeats is employing the conventional pastoral opposition between the *urbs ingrata* or "ungrateful city" and the countryside, but rethought along Irish cultural lines as an opposition between Britain and (western) Ireland.[11] In *At the Hawk's Well*, the characters are never there to see this water; somehow, they always miss it. Yeats sympathised with the protagonist: for Cuchulain, missing out on the flood inspired his heroism. Synge's sardonic play ironises this in the very different motives of the Douls' rejection of the healing well-water.

[11] I am grateful to Alex Davis for making this point.

There is no cure at all in the play, not even at the end; the glory and beauty that are present are represented in continuous struggle. There is a profoundly personal slant to the dramatic piece. Both Yeats's and Synge's plays express a kind of wearied scepticism in relation to bubbling well-water that begs some uncomfortable questions. The Revival promises a new Ireland and a new world, but could this be achieved and, if it could, how desirable would this be?

* * *

Synge and Yeats experiment with blindness in a similar way in their writing. An extract from *At the Hawk's Well* indicates that Yeats had a passage from Synge's *The Well of the Saints* in his mind when he composed his own play. In *At the Hawk's Well*, when the old and young man hear "[*t*]*he Guardian of the Well*" who wears a hawk mask and "*gives the cry of the hawk*," the young man considers the risk of blindness (line 146). Cuchulain says:

> It sounded like the sudden cry of a hawk,
> But there's no wing in sight. As I came hither
> A *great grey hawk* swept down out of the sky,
> And though I have good hawks, the best in the world
> I had fancied, I have not seen its like. It flew
> As though it would have torn me with its beak,
> Or *blinded me*, smiting with that great wing. (lines 148–54; emphases added)

Likewise, Timmy uses a simile involving a hawk to depict accurate eyesight in *The Well of the Saints*: "Ay, a fine saint, who's going round through the churches of Ireland, with a long cloak on him, and naked feet, for he's brought a sup of the water slung at his side, and, with the like of him, any little drop is enough to cure the dying, or to *make the blind see as clear as the grey hawks* do be high up, on a still day, sailing the sky" (81; act 1; emphasis added). In Yeats's play, hawks are associated with inducing blindness; however, Synge links hawks to clear vision. This forms a subtle conversation between both writers about the vision for the Irish Revival. Yeats's "great grey hawk" that "flew / As though it would have torn me with its beak, / Or blinded me, smiting with that great wing" is a frightening prospect in comparison to Synge's more passive "grey hawks" that have "clear" eyesight and are "sailing the sky." For Synge's characters, the threat of blindness is not a threat to them at all, and so the predatory and harmful capacities of hawks are not feared. The fear of hawks is traceable in Yeats's *The Countess Cathleen* (1892) when Cathleen describes a "blinding" storm and remarks, "I know what clamour frighted them—some bird, / Some hawk or kestrel, chased its prey to this" (lines 883, 801–02). Gregory also adds to this conversation about hawks and their harmful abilities. In "Book Five: Great Wonders of the Olden Time" in *Saints and Wonders* (1907), a collection of accounts from the Irish people about saints and their miracles, Gregory writes about a destructive hawk—a bird of prey known for hunting and stealing smaller animals—that parallels the hawks in both Yeats's and Synge's work. St. Ciaran heals the damage that is done by the hawk:

> The first of the saints to be born in Ireland of the saints was Ciaran, that was of the blood of the nobles of Leinster. And the first of the wonders he did was in the island of Cleire, and he but a young child at the time. There came a hawk in the air over his head, and it stooped down before him and took up a little bird that was sitting on a nest. And pity for the little bird came on Ciaran and it was bad to him the way it was. And the hawk turned back and left the bird before him, and it half dead and trembling; and Ciaran bade it to rise up and it rose and went up safe and well to its nest, by the grace of God. It was Patrick bade Ciaran after that to go to the Well of Uaran, the mering where the north meets with the south in the middle part of Ireland. (127)

With earnestness and sincerity, her writing style praises St. Ciaran's healing; Gregory accepts his honourable reasons to heal the bird and she does not question his motives. Gregory, unlike Synge, treats the healing wells with a profound respect for both the saints associated with them as well as their important role in Irish life. For both Yeats and Gregory, perhaps hawks represent the violence and tensions and conflicts and contradictions that pose a threat to Ireland's overall health and the success of the Revival. Synge, however, instead befriends these clear-sighted hawks that can inflict blindness on others; he seems to believe that health and revival could be found in illness and anti-revival.

Synge experiments with the homonyms of "well" as both a source of healing water and a health state; he then rejects physical wellness in exchange for a subjective "wellness." Martin Doul, for example, chooses blindness so that he does not have to work in the blacksmith's forge and can wander around living off charity that is given to him by passers-by on the road. Synge uses this image as a microcosm of the Congested Districts Board, which phased out traditional Irish styles of working and instead imposed set modern occupations designed to modernise and progress the areas at the expense of originality and uniqueness. To Synge, however, healing water from the west is an ambiguous substance, and its representation is a way of questioning both the Irish Revival and the homogenising capacities of modernity.

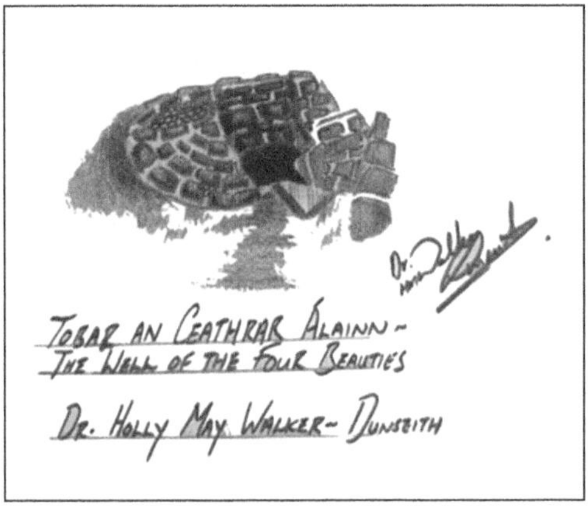

Tobar an Ceathrar Álainn—The Well of the Four Beauties

CHAPTER 8

Conclusion

The three key Revivalists—Yeats, Gregory, and Synge—all took different approaches to traditional medicine in their works. Of the three, Yeats's approach to medicine is the most consciously metaphorical, as he explores Ireland's revival back to health. Gregory, on the other hand, is more interested in the literal practice of herbal medicine, and she devoted considerable time both to practitioners and to their remedies. Synge is a special case. He is much more interested in anti-health, and this is evident in his play *The Well of the Saints*, which links the powers of the healing well with the ubiquitous powers of utilitarian and capitalist modernity in order to question the latter. Nevertheless, despite Synge's familiarity with and closeness to illness in both his fiction and personal life, there is no doubt that he still acknowledges traditional medicine and its place in national life, albeit in a troubling manner. Traditional medicine is both a *topos* in Revival-era work and a metaphor for writing at a critical point in the history of modern Ireland.

For Yeats, *The Wanderings of Oisin* is an allegory of strength and weakness, and Yeats depicts recoveries from age, illness, and decrepitude to renewed strength. The poem's title, layout, content, rhythm, and line lengths are all germane to the theme of "wandering," and both visually and metaphorically demonstrate this concept. "Wandering" had been seen as a weakness. Witness Patrick's admonition to the aged Oisin that he is "wandering" in his "mind"—but Yeats recasts it as a resource and source

H. M. Walker-Dunseith, *Traditional Medicine in the Irish Literary Revival*, New Directions in Irish and Irish American Literature,
https://doi.org/10.1007/978-3-031-82459-3_8

of strength: a means by which Ireland will regain the flexibility to recover and follow a wandering path to recovery (*VP* line 2). Several years later, Yeats first wandered the area around Coole-Ballylee, collecting the broken fragments of Irish folklore and building them into a new indigenous body. Reclaiming wandering from a medical sign of weakness to a restorative quality of the spirit was an important part of Yeats's project. It was something that could be brought from the Land of the Young to a debilitated present-day Ireland. He was to find his real-life Tír na nÓg at Thoor Ballylee.

Yeats's tower is a place of healing and renewal on a personal and national level. Biddy Early is the connective tissue that links folklore and medicine. Through their contact with her healing moss, the millboards with which Yeats restored the tower carry with them magical and salutary associations. Lady Wilde's collection of cures, as read by Yeats himself, represents moss as a therapeutic and magical substance in Irish folklore. Thoor Ballylee is not the only thing those millboards "cured"; just as Yeats patches up the tower, he simultaneously patches together the world's wounds. A practitioner in words rather than medicine, Yeats rebuilds Thoor Ballylee as an amalgamation of fractures that might, in being re-set, heal stronger. He fixes together national and international conflict as well as remedy the wider tensions at the heart of the Irish Revival: between Irish and English, the ancient and the new, the mystical and the scientific.

Elizabeth Outka has, like my work, investigated the medical contexts of Yeats's poetry. Her book *Viral Modernism: The Influenza Pandemic and Interwar Literature* (2019) "investigates a modernist mystery: why does the deadly 1918-1919 influenza pandemic seem to make so few appearances in British, Irish, and American literature of the period?" (1). She writes, "In November 1918, at the height of the pandemic's deadly second wave, W. B. Yeats watched helplessly as his pregnant wife, George, struggled to fight off the virus at their rented house in Dublin" (167). Outka clearly shows that this experience of serious illness correlates with the fact that "[j]ust a few weeks later, during his wife's recovery, Yeats wrote arguably his most famous poem, 'The Second Coming,'" which "was not only completed while the pandemic was still unfolding but written directly after witnessing a near-fatal case [i.e. his wife's near-death]" (167). She notices that "[t]he focus on the poem's political violence has obscured, however, the distinct viral violence that was unfolding at the same time, both within Yeats's home and in the streets of Dublin" (168).

Outka's work shows that the health contexts of Irish literature, for so long neglected, are now gaining attention.

Augusta Gregory completed her ten-year transformation as a new woman with a fresh vision for her life. She fostered a deliberate selective memory and self-selective process, which enabled her to forget her past and become a spiritual self-portrait of Cathleen Ni Houlihan and a medical mirror image of Biddy Early. Based on the rejuvenated *cailleach* and the folk healer, Gregory put into practice a new life that focussed on reviving Ireland, restoring the health of her neighbourhood, and challenging colonialism. Ó Crualaoich's identification of the *cailleach* as a healer that can offer different well-being services provides a new angle with which to view this traditional Irish character. Gregory, too, had a multi-faceted identity. As a *bean ghlúine* or midwife, she brought a revived Ireland into the world; as a *bean feasa* or wise woman, she mixed medicines for her neighbours. Her ideas of her own rejuvenation and that of Ireland were inextricably linked together.

Gregory also took herbal medicine into her own hands, both literally and in literature. At the same time as Gregory was innovating a new literary language based on her locality in the west of Ireland, she created a symbolic language of healing herbs. Her folkloric explorations, specifically in relation to herbs, formed a foundation for her entire literary career and gave her a form of communication that could reach a wide audience. Whilst Gregory did not get a chance to fully root the herbs in *The Pot of Broth*, due to the tramp not fitting into a healing role, she later planted the herbs in more suitable soil, her collection titled *Visions and Beliefs in the West of Ireland* (1920) and her play named *The Golden Apple: A Play for Kiltartan Children* (1916), and was able to reap more benefits from her many years of collecting folklore. Her early collaborative works with Yeats gave her time to gather and think about how she would use the herbs in a solo work. By writing *Poets and Dreamers* and *Visions and Beliefs*, Gregory provided a delayed acknowledgement for her herbalism teacher Ruane and brought her knowledge of healing and cures into the compass of the Irish Revival. Both Gregory and Yeats strived to benefit Ireland as a nation, and the world.

Recent scholarship on Gregory includes Siobhán Purcell's article titled "Beckett and Disability Biopolitics: The Case of Cuchulain" (2019). Through this article, Purcell seeks to bring health and disability into Irish studies. Purcell writes, "In his depiction of the hero Cuchulain, Samuel Beckett interrogates how disability and compulsory able-bodiedness are foundational myths for the Irish Free State" (52). Referring to Marion Quirici's work on disability in Irish literature,[1] Purcell states that "[t]his association of the Celtic body with disability and lameness inflects the foundational myths that represent a new type of Irish body" and "[a]s Quirici has demonstrated, Yeats and Lady Gregory's *Cathleen ni Houlihan* epitomises this examination of the body politic and couches it squarely in terms of impairment and disability" (55). Purcell writes about ableist themes and Quirici focusses on ability versus disability. I have added to this discussion the argument that Cathleen Ni Houlihan is a role model, alongside healers Biddy Early and Bridget Ruane, that allows her to explore her own Irishness and leave behind her colonial associations. Her pedagogical encounter with Bridget Ruane led her to practising herbal medicine using herbs from her own garden, such as the juniper that she used to make the forester's panacea remedy. I discovered that, based on her reading material and the ingredients available in her garden, Gregory was likely to have mixed this specific remedy. Her literary meeting with Biddy Early, both from written accounts and spoken testimonies from the people around her, also encouraged her to write herbs into both her prose and plays. This herbal content, which she sought herself, helped her to transition from collaborative to independent work and gave her the freedom, not only to mix her own remedies, but also to concoct her own fiction.

Synge was more interested in anti-health and anti-Revival rather than wellness and strength as a theme. Traditional healing practices are at the heart of Synge's *The Well of the Saints*, as a character named the Saint travels Ireland with its healing waters. However, the waters' curative powers are not universally welcomed: the play's protagonists, Martin and Mary Doul, ultimately reject the gift of sight. Though this seems inexplicable, Synge's ideas regarding the nature of modernity and development make this outcome inevitable. He ironically and irreverently uses the character of the Saint to represent the charitable impulse that might provide people with what they need—sight—but not what they want. Synge employs "sight" as a concept that distinguishes eyesight from mindsight, objective from subjective perspectives, and this confirms his view of well-being as separate from good physical health. Gregory, unlike Synge, treats the healing wells with a profound respect for both the saints associated with them as well as their important role in Irish life. To Synge, however, healing

[1] See Matthew Arnold's *On the Study of Celtic Literature* (1867) and Marion Quirici's "*Cathleen ni Houlihan* and the Disability Aesthetics of Irish National Culture" (2015).

water from the west is an ambiguous substance, and its representation is a way of questioning both the Irish Revival and the homogenising capacities of modernity.

In 2021, Seán Hewitt published *J. M. Synge: Nature, Politics, Modernism*. In the introduction, he writes, "This study thus charts the development of Synge's modernist art as a fraught reactive battle between aesthetic socialism and the increasing pressures of capitalist modernization and restrictive political nationalism" (5). Further on in the introduction, he notes the importance of the national body's rejuvenation to the notion of Revival and recognises a language of regeneration that spans throughout Synge's works (8).[2] In reference to some health-related topics in Synge's "The Oppression of the Hills" in *In Wicklow, West Kerry and Connemara*, Hewitt argues that "[i]n such passages, Wicklow becomes contrary to the virtues of vitality and health that Synge prized in the peasantry" (65). In relation to *The Well of the Saints*, Hewitt comments, "As in Synge's depiction of the relief workers in his articles 'From the Congested Districts' [in *In Wicklow, West Kerry and Connemara*] …, degradation is seen to ensue from the imposition of an unnatural life on the 'natural' peasantry" (133). Hewitt concludes that Synge's "trajectory towards modernism, and his characteristic irony and undercutting of Romanticism, are symptomatic of the tension between the political pressures of his Ireland (and of literary Revivalism) and his own aesthetic and philosophical values" and that "[o]ver his career, as his own political and social consciousness developed in nuance, this fundamental conflict became more pressing, and led him to the production of a literature which was as much a form of artistic as political protest" (211). In my book, I have explored the healing qualities of wells, their presence in Ireland, and accounts of people being cured using the water from these wells. In addition, I have found a link between Synge's asthmatic congestion and the suggested "congestion" of the population in the Congested Districts, and I have evaluated the influence of Synge's personal health in his writing. Furthermore, I have discovered that Synge used the word "well" as a homonym for both a literal "well" in

[2] In Hewitt's book, he includes a footnote at this sentence, quoting from Joep Leerssen's *Remembrance and Imagination: Patterns in the Historical and Literary Representation of Ireland in the Nineteenth Century* (1996): "The horizon of expectation of the Abbey audiences was habituated, through a thousand turns of phrase and metaphor, to see Irish cultural nationalism as aiming at a *revival*, a *rejuvenation*, turning Kathleen Ní Houlihan from an old hag into a young queen" (Leerssen, 222; qtd. in Hewitt, 8).

Inishmore and the abstract concept of "wellness," which sets up a wider tension between objective and subjective morality in his play.

Yeats, Gregory, and Synge used traditional medicine as metaphor in their literary works, at times gesturing towards the possibility that Ireland was a culture and nation in the act of healing itself, and at times questioning these nationalist discourses. Their respective uses of traditional medicine and cures help to root their works in the Irish countryside and its folk culture. In their works, cures and traditional medicine allow them to approach the idea of bodily health both as subject and as metaphor. By depicting healers, herbs and other cures, these writers, sometimes, raise hopeful ideas of a wider renewal.

Bibliography

Primary Sources

I. Accounts and Reports

Congested Districts Board for Ireland. *First Annual Report of the Congested Districts Board for Ireland*. Alex Thom, 1893.

Royal Commission on Labour. *The Agricultural Labourer: Ireland: Reports: Part 1*. Vol. 4 of *The Agricultural Labourer*. Her Majesty's Stationery Office / Eyre and Spottiswoode, 1893.

The Schools' Manuscript Collection. NFCS 0138D: "Ailments" 34–37; Kate Hastings, Leenavesta, County Mayo. Collector: Caitlín Ní Oistín, St. Bridget's (school), Derrymore, County Mayo, 5 April 1938. Teacher: Máire Uí hOistín. The Schools' Manuscript Collection, National Folklore Collection, U College Dublin, Dublin. Online Manuscript. *National Folklore Collection*, www.duchas.ie/en/cbes/5215813/5215332.

———. *NFCS* 0596: "Biddy Early" 126–27; James Meaney, Creevagh More, County Clare. Collector: Mary O'Loughlin, An Daingean, Cuinche (school), Dangan, County Clare, 1 April 1938–30 June 1938. Teachers: Stiofán Mac Clúin and Treasa Ní Chonmara. The Schools' Manuscript Collection, National Folklore Collection, U College Dublin, Dublin. Online Manuscript. *National Folklore Collection*, www.duchas.ie/en/cbes/5177641/5175691.

H. M. Walker-Dunseith, *Traditional Medicine in the Irish Literary Revival*, New Directions in Irish and Irish American Literature,
https://doi.org/10.1007/978-3-031-82459-3

———. *NFCS* 0591: "Biddy Early" 272; Mrs. John Powell, collector's mother, parent, Kilbarron, County Clare. Collector: Prionnsias Mac Giolla Phóil, Anach Néill (school), Annaghneal, County Clare, 11 January 1939–31 January 1938. Teacher: B. B. Uí Dhonnchadha. The Schools' Manuscript Collection, National Folklore Collection, U College Dublin, Dublin. Online Manuscript. *National Folklore Collection*, www.duchas.ie/en/cbes/5177625/5173913/5199488.

———. *NFCS* 0107: 250–52; Collector's father, parent, Holywell Lower, Ballyhaunis, County Mayo. Collector: Paddy O'Brien, Scoil Mhuire, Béal Átha hAmhnais (school), Ballyhaunis, County Mayo, c. 1937–1939. Teacher: S. T. Ó Maolagáin. The Schools' Manuscript Collection, National Folklore Collection, U College Dublin, Dublin. Online Manuscript. *National Folklore Collection*, www.duchas.ie/en/cbes/4427885/4354373.

———. *NFCS* 0732: "Cures" 401–08; Collector: Maureen Hurley, Kilbeggan (Mercy Convent) (school), Kilbeggan, County Westmeath, January 1938–January 1939. Teacher: Sr Philomena. The Schools' Manuscript Collection, National Folklore Collection, U College Dublin, Dublin. Online Manuscript. *National Folklore Collection*, www.duchas.ie/en/cbes/5009069/4983414/5120081.

———. *NFCS* 0751: "A Funny Story" 85–86; Mrs. Gerety (32), Gorteenclareen, County Longford. Collector: Teresa Gerety, Gurteen, Ballymahon [school], Gorteenclareen, County Longford. 22 November 1937—19 December 1938. Teacher: T. Ó. Murchadha. The Schools' Manuscript Collection, National Folklore Collection, U College Dublin, Dublin. Online Manuscript. *National Folklore Collection*, www.duchas.ie/en/cbes/5009140/4990587/5100310.

———. *NFCS* 0847: "Herb Cures" 91–95; Bridget Doran (50). Collector: Patrick Galavan, The Rower (B.), Inistioge (school), County Kilkenny, October 1937 – 20 December 1938. Teacher: Risteárd Ó Cuirrín. The Schools' Manuscript Collection, National Folklore Collection, U College Dublin, Dublin. Online Manuscript. *National Folklore Collection*, www.duchas.ie/en/cbes/4758506/4749788.

———. *NFCS* 1019: "Herbs" 174–75; Collector: Minnie Moore, Benbawn (school), Binbane, County Cavan, c. 1937–1939. Teacher: M. Gillespie. The Schools' Manuscript Collection, National Folklore Collection, U College Dublin, Dublin. Online Manuscript. *National Folklore Collection*, www.duchas.ie/en/cbes/5070836/5068904/5099175.

———. *NFCS* 0050: "How Biddy Early Got Her Charms" 157; Mrs. Henry, grandparent, Gorteenboy, County Galway. Collector: Bernard Regan, Réidh Reamhar (school), Reyrawer, County Galway, c. 1937–1939. Teacher: Seán A. Mac Fhloinn. The Schools' Manuscript Collection, National Folklore Collection, U College Dublin, Dublin. Online Manuscript. *National Folklore Collection*, www.duchas.ie/en/cbes/4583308/4578395/4587825.

———. *NFCS* 0722: "Local Cures" 110–12; Collector: Helen Cooney, Carpenterstown (Templefanum) (school), Carpenterstown, County Westmeath, c. 1937–1939. Teacher: Mary Smyth. The Schools' Manuscript Collection, National Folklore Collection, U College Dublin, Dublin. Online Manuscript. *National Folklore Collection*, www.duchas.ie/en/cbes/5009034/4979325.

———. *NFCS* 0845: "Local Cures" 233–34; James Cullen (c. 60), Smartscastle West, County Kilkenny. Collector: Strang's Mills, Kilmacow (school), Strangsmill, County Kilkenny, January 1938–January 1939. Teacher: Richard Rellis. The Schools' Manuscript Collection, National Folklore Collection, U College Dublin, Dublin. Online Manuscript. *National Folklore Collection*, www.duchas.ie/en/cbes/4758499/4748961/4786591.

———. *NFCS* 0865: "Local Cures" 510–15; Collector: Maire Horgan (12), Clinstown (school), County Kilkenny, c. 1937–1939. Teacher: S. Ó Dúnlaing. The Schools' Manuscript Collection, National Folklore Collection, U College Dublin, Dublin. Online Manuscript. *National Folklore Collection*, www.duchas.ie/en/cbes/4758578/4756220.

———. *NFCS* 0800: "Local Cures: Wild-Fire or Fever" 153–60; Clonbulloge [school], Clonbulloge, County Offaly, 20 June 1938–27 June 1938. Teacher: A. Fitzgerald. The Schools' Manuscript Collection, National Folklore Collection, U College Dublin, Dublin. Online Manuscript. *National Folklore Collection*, www.duchas.ie/en/cbes/5044568/5023102/5143446.

———. *NFCS* 1059: "Luibheanna" 59–62; Muiris Ó hUiginn (72), Ardara, County Donegal. Collector: Pádraic Ó Breisleáin, An Mhín Mhór (school), Meenmore, County Donegal, 1932. Teacher: Pádraic Ó Breisleáin. The Schools' Manuscript Collection, National Folklore Collection, U College Dublin, Dublin. Online Manuscript. *National Folklore Collection*, www.duchas.ie/en/cbes/4428367/4400591.

———. *NFCS* 0904: "The Magic Apples" 126; teacher; Collector: Mary Kennedy, Baile Uí Mhurchadha, Borris, Ballymurphy, County Carlow, October 1937–December 1938. Teacher: Michael Ó Seachnasaigh. The Schools' Manuscript Collection, National Folklore Collection, U College Dublin, Dublin. Online Manuscript. *National Folklore Collection*, www.duchas.ie/en/cbes/5044664/5030226/5141541.

II. Autobiographies, Biographies, Diaries, Journals, and Memoirs

Foster, R. F. *The Apprentice Mage, 1865-1914.* Oxford UP, 1997. Vol. 1 of *W. B. Yeats: A Life.*

———. *The Apprentice Mage. The Arch-Poet, 1915-1939.* Oxford UP, 2003. Vol. 2 of *W. B. Yeats: A Life.*

Gregory, Augusta. *Coole: Completed from the Manuscript.* Edited by Colin Smythe, Dolmen P, 1971.

———. *Lady Gregory's Diaries, 1892-1902.* Edited by James Pethica, Colin Smythe, 1996.

———. *Lady Gregory's Journals, 1916-1930.* Edited by Lennox Robinson, Putnam, 1946.

———. *Seventy Years: Being the Autobiography of Lady Gregory.* Edited by Colin Smythe, Macmillan, 1976.

Johnson, James. *Change of Air; or, the Diary of a Philosopher in Pursuit of Health and Recreation.* S. Highley, 1831.

McCormack, W. J. *Fool of the Family: A Life of J. M. Synge.* New York UP, 2000.

Nic Shiubhlaigh, Máire. *The Splendid Years: Recollections of Maire Nic Shiubhlaigh.* Edited by Edward Kenny, James Duffy, 1955.

Synge, John Millington. *Autobiography of J. M. Synge: Constructed from the Manuscripts.* Edited by Alan Price, Dolmen P / Oxford UP, 1965.

Tóibín, Colm. *Lady Gregory's Toothbrush.* Picador, 2003.

Tynan, Katharine. *The Middle Years.* Constable, 1916.

Yeats, William Butler. *Autobiographies.* Edited by William H. O'Donnell and Douglas N. Archibald, Scribner, 1999. Vol. 3 of *The Collected Works of W. B. Yeats.*

———. *Memoirs.* Edited by Denis Donoghue, Macmillan, 1973.

III. Letters

Yeats, William Butler. *The Collected Letters of W. B. Yeats, 1865-1895.* Edited by John Kelly and Eric Domville. Vol. 1, Clarendon P, 1986.

———. *The Collected Letters of W. B. Yeats, 1901-1904.* Edited by John Kelly and Ronald Schuchard, 1994. Vol. 3, Clarendon P, 1994.

———. *The Letters of W. B. Yeats.* Edited by Allan Wade. Rupert Hart-Davis, 1954.

———. *Letters to Katharine Tynan.* Edited by Roger McHugh. Clonmore and Reynolds, 1953.

Yeats, William Butler and T. Sturge Moore. *W. B. Yeats and T. Sturge Moore: Their Correspondence, 1901-1937.* Edited by Ursula Bridge. Oxford UP, 1953.

IV. Plays

Gregory, Augusta. *Selected Plays of Lady Gregory.* Edited by Mary FitzGerald, Colin Smythe / Catholic U of America P, 1993. Vol. 3 of *Irish Drama Selections.*

Synge, John Millington. *Plays: Book I.* Edited by Ann Saddlemyer, Colin Smythe / Catholic U of America P, 1968. Vol. 3 of *J. M. Synge: Collected Works.*

———. *Plays: Book II*. Edited by Ann Saddlemyer, Oxford UP, 1968. Vol. 4 of *J. M. Synge: Collected Works*.

Yeats, William Butler and Augusta Gregory. *Collaborative One-Act Plays, 1901-1903: Cathleen ni Houlihan, The Pot of Broth, The Country of the Young, Heads or Harps: Manuscript Materials*. Edited by James Pethica, Cornell UP, 2006.

Yeats, William Butler. *The Countess Kathleen and Various Legends and Lyrics*. T. Fisher Unwin, 1892.

———. *The Hour-Glass and Other Plays*. Macmillan, 1904. Vol. 2 of *Plays for an Irish Theatre*.

———. *The Hour-Glass, Cathleen ni Houlihan, The Pot of Broth*. A. H. Bullen, 1904. Vol. 2 of *Plays for an Irish Theatre*.

———. *The Hour-Glass, Cathleen ni Houlihan, The Pot of Broth*. Maunsel, 1905.

———. *The Variorum Edition of the Plays of W. B. Yeats*. Edited by Russell K. Alspach, assisted by Catharine C. Alspach, Macmillan, 1966.

V. Poetry

AE [George William Russell]. *Collected Poems*. Macmillan, 1913.

Ancient and Modern Scottish Songs, Heroic Ballads, Etc. Collected from Memory, Tradition, and Ancient Authors. Vol. 2. John Wotherspoon / James Dickson and Charles Elliot, 1776.

Coimín, Micheál. *Laoi Oisín ar Tír na n-Óg: The Lay of Oisín in the Land of Youth*. Translated by Tomás Ó Flannghaile, M. H. Gill, 1896.

Duffy, Charles Gavan, editor. *The Ballad Poetry of Ireland*. James Duffy, 1845.

Gregory, Lady Augusta. *The Kiltartan Poetry Book: Prose Translations from the Irish*. G. P. Putnam's Sons / The Knickerbocker P, 1919.

Hogan, Michael. *Lays and Legends of Thomond, with Historical and Traditional Notes*. M. H. Gill and Son, 1880.

Jeffares, A. Norman. *A Commentary on the Collected Poems of W. B. Yeats*. Palgrave Macmillan, 1968.

Keats, John. *The Complete Poetical Works and Letters of John Keats*. Houghton, Mifflin, 1899.

MacDonagh, Thomas. *Literature in Ireland: Studies Irish and Anglo-Irish*. Talbot P, 1916.

Macpherson, James. *The Works of Ossian, the Son of Fingal*. 3rd ed., T. Becket and P. A. Dehondt, 1765. 2 vols.

O'Rahilly, Egan. *Dánta Aodagáin Uí Rataille: The Poems of Egan O'Rahilly*. Edited by Patrick S. Dinneen and Tadhg O'Donoghue, Irish Texts Society / David Nutt, 1911. Vol. 3 of *Irish Texts Society*.

Virgil. *An English Version of the Eclogues of Virgil*. Translated by Samuel Palmer, Seeley, 1883.

———. *The Fourth Georgic of Virgil, Containing an Account of the Treatment of Bees, the Story of Aristaeus and His Bees, the Episode of Orpheus and Eurydice; and an Article on the Gladiators.* Translated by R. M. Millington, Longmans, Green, Reader, and Dyer, 1870.

Wilde, Jane. *Poems by Speranza.* James Duffy, 1864.

Yeats, William Butler. *Early Poems and Stories.* Macmillan, 1925.

———. *Michael Robartes and the Dancer: Manuscript Materials.* Edited by Thomas Parkinson and Anne Brannen, Cornell UP, 1994.

———. *Poems.* T. Fisher Unwin, 1895.

———. *Poems.* T. Fisher Unwin, 1899.

———. *Poems.* T. Fisher Unwin, 1901.

———. *The Variorum Edition of the Poems of W. B. Yeats.* Edited by Peter Allt and Russell K. Alspach, Macmillan, 1957.

———. *The Wanderings of Oisin and Other Poems.* Kegan Paul, 1889.

VI. Prose

Blake, William. *The Marriage of Heaven and Hell.* J. W. Luce, 1906.

Blunt, Anne. *Pilgrimage to Nejd.* Edited by William Scawen Blunt, vol. 1, John Murray, 1881.

Cath Maige Tuired: The Second Battle of Mag Tuired. Translated by Elizabeth A. Gray, Irish Texts Society, No. 52, 1982. *CELT: Corpus of Electronic Texts,* celt.ucc.ie/published/T300010/.

Dickens, Charles. *Great Expectations.* Vol. 2, Chapman and Hall, 1861.

Gregory, Lady Augusta. *Cuchulain of Muirthemne: The Story of the Men of the Red Branch of Ulster.* John Murray, 1903.

———. *A Book of Saints and Wonders Put Down Here by Lady Gregory According to the Old Writings and the Memory of the People of Ireland.* Charles Scribner's Sons, 1907.

———. *Gods and Fighting Men: The Story of the Tuatha de Danaan and of the Fianna of Ireland.* John Murray, 1904.

———. *Poets and Dreamers: Studies and Translations from the Irish.* Hodges, Figgis / John Murray, 1903.

———. *Visions and Beliefs in the West of Ireland.* G. P. Putnam's Sons, 1920. 2 vols.

Heaney, Seamus. *Finders Keepers: Selected Prose, 1971-2001.* Faber and Faber, 2002.

Joyce, James. *Dubliners.* Wordsworth, 2001.

———. *Ulysses.* John Rodker, 1922.

Reynolds, James. *Ghosts in Irish Houses.* Bonanza Books, 1947.

Synge, John Millington. *Prose.* Edited by Alan Price, Colin Smythe / Catholic U of America P, 1982. Vol. 2 of *J. M. Synge: Collected Works.*

Tolstoy, Leo. *Anna Karenina.* Edited by Gary Saul Morson, translated by Marian Schwartz, Yale UP, 2014.

Wilde, Lady Jane. *Ancient Cures, Charms, and Usages of Ireland*. Ward and Downey, 1890.
———. *Ancient Legends, Mystic Charms, and Superstitions of Ireland*. Ticknor, 1887. 2 vols.
Yeats, William Butler. *Fairy and Folk Tales of the Irish Peasantry*. Walter Scott, 1888.
———. *The Irish Dramatic Movement*. Edited by Mary FitzGerald and Richard J. Finneran, Scribner, 2003. Vol. 8 of *The Collected Works of W. B. Yeats*.
———. *Mythologies*. Edited by Warwick Gould and Deirdre Toomey, Palgrave Macmillan, 2005.
———. *Uncollected Prose*. Edited by John P. Frayne and Colton Johnson, vol. 2, Columbia UP, 1975.

Secondary Sources

VII. Books

Arkins, Brian. *Builders of My Soul: Greek and Roman Themes in Yeats*. Colin Smythe, 1990.
Arnold, Matthew. *On the Study of Celtic Literature*. Smith, Elder, 1867.
Bauer, William Waldo. *Potions, Remedies, and Old Wives' Tales*. Doubleday, 1969.
Breathnach, Ciara. *The Congested Districts Board of Ireland, 1891-1923: Poverty and Development in the West of Ireland*. Four Courts P, 2005.
Bruna, Giulia. *J. M. Synge and Travel Writing of the Irish Revival*. Syracuse UP, 2017.
Bryant, Sophie. *Celtic Ireland*. Kegan Paul, Trench, 1889.
Carroll, Marion and John Scally. *My Miracle Cure: An Extraordinary Story of Hope, Healing and the Power of Faith*. Bonnier Books, 2021.
Catalogue of Printed Books Formerly at the Library at Coole. Sotheby, 1972.
Clark, Katharine. *An Irish Book of Shadows: Tuatha De Danann*. Galde P, 2001.
Crowley, John., William J. Smyth, and Mike Murphy. *Atlas of the Great Irish Famine*. Cork UP, 2012.
Culpeper, Nicholas. *The Complete Herbal*. Thomas Kelly, 1835.
Dalyrmple, William. *The Anarchy: The Relentless Rise of the East India Company*. Bloomsbury, 2020.
Dillane, Fionnuala, Naomi McAreavey, and Emilie Pine. *The Body in Pain in Irish Literature and Culture*. Palgrave Macmillan; Springer Nature, 2016.
Drabble, Margaret, et al., editors. *The Concise Oxford Companion to English Literature*. 3rd ed., Oxford UP, 2007.
Evelyn, John. *Silva: or, A Discourse of Forest-Trees*. A. Ward, 1786. 2 vols.

Falci, Eric. *Continuity and Change in Irish Poetry, 1966-2010.* Cambridge UP, 2012.

Farmar, Tony. *Patients, Potions and Physicians: A Social History of Medicine in Ireland.* A. & A. Farmar, 2004.

Fletcher, Guy. *The Routledge Handbook of Philosophy of Well-Being.* Routledge, 2017.

Folkard, Richard. *Plant Lore, Legends, and Lyrics: Embracing the Myths, Traditions, Superstitions, and Folk-lore of the Plant Kingdom.* Sampson Low, Marston, Searle, and Rivington, 1884.

Foster, John Wilson. *Fictions of the Irish Literary Revival: A Changeling Art.* Syracuse UP / Gill and Macmillan, 1987.

Foucault, Michel. *The Birth of the Clinic: An Archaeology of Medical Perception.* Translated by A. M. Sheridan Smith, Vintage Books, 1975.

Hanley, Mary D. *Thoor Ballylee—Home of William Butler Yeats.* Edited by Liam Miller, Dolmen P, 1965.

Harmon, Maurice. *Austin Clarke, 1896-1974: A Critical Introduction.* Wolfhound, 1989.

Hewitt, Seán. *J. M. Synge: Nature, Politics, Modernism.* Oxford UP, 2021.

The Holy Bible. Revised Standard Version: Second Catholic Edition. Ascension Publishing, 2018.

Howe, LeAnne and Padraig Kirwan. *Famine Pots: The Choctaw-Irish Gift Exchange, 1847-Present.* Michigan State UP, 2020.

Hynes, Eugene. *Knock: The Virgin's Apparition in Nineteenth-Century Ireland.* Cork UP, 2017.

Kearney, Gerry. *The Persse Family of County Galway: Genealogy and History, 1554-1964.* Gerry Kearney, 2016.

Kiberd, Declan and P. J. Mathews. *The Handbook of the Irish Revival: An Anthology of Irish Cultural and Political Writings, 1891-1922.* Notre U of Notre Dame P, 2016.

Kohfeldt, Mary Lou. *Lady Gregory: The Woman Behind the Irish Renaissance.* André Deutsch, 1985.

Larrissy, Edward. *Yeats the Poet: The Measures of Difference.* Harvester Wheatsheaf, 1994.

Leitch, Vincent B., editor. *The Norton Anthology of Theory and Criticism.* Norton, 2001.

Lee, Joseph. *The Modernisation of Irish Society, 1848-1918.* Gill and Macmillan, 1989.

Leerssen, Joep. *Remembrance and Imagination: Patterns in the Historical and Literary Representation of Ireland in the Nineteenth Century.* Cork UP, 1996.

Logan, Patrick. *Making the Cure: A Look at Irish Folk Medicine.* Talbot P, 1972.

———. *The Holy Wells of Ireland.* Colin Smythe, 1992.

Longenbach, James. *Stone Cottage: Pound, Yeats, and Modernism.* Oxford UP, 1988.

Mattar, Sinéad Garrigan. *Primitivism, Science, and the Irish Revival.* Oxford UP, 2004.

Miller, Ian. *Reforming Food in Post-Famine Ireland: Medicine, Science and Improvement, 1845-1922.* Manchester UP, 2014.

Miller, Philip. *The Gardener's and Botanist's Dictionary.* F. C. and J. Rivington et al. / Law and Gilbert, 1807.

Mill, John Stuart. *Utilitarianism.* Longmans, Green, 1879.

Mitchell, Thomas Duché. *Materia Medica and Therapeutics.* Lippincott, Grambo, 1850.

Moore, Ronnie and Stuart McClean. *Folk Healing and Health Care Practices in Britain and Ireland: Stethoscopes, Wands and Crystals.* Berghahn Books, 2010.

New York Public Library. *Bulletin of The New York Public Library: Astor, Lenox and Tilden Foundations.* Vol. 72, New York Public Library, 1968.

Nunn, Joan. *Fashion in Costume, 1200-1980.* Schocken Books, 1984.

Ó Crualaoich, Gearóid. *The Book of the Cailleach: Stories of the Wise-Woman Healer.* Cork UP, 2017.

Ó Gráda, Cormac. *The Great Irish Famine.* Cambridge UP, 1995. Issue 7 of *New Studies in Economic and Social History.*

O'Shea, Edward. *A Descriptive Catalog of W. B. Yeats' Library.* Garland Publishing, 1985.

O'Toole, Fintan. *A History of Ireland in 100 Objects.* Royal Irish Academy, 2013.

Outka, Elizabeth. *Viral Modernism: The Influenza Pandemic and Interwar Literature.* Columbia UP, 2019.

Pettigrew, Thomas Joseph. *On Superstitions Connected with the History and the Practice of Medicine and Surgery.* Ed. Barrington and Geo. D. Haswell, 1844.

Raine, Kathleen. *Yeats the Initiate: Essays on Certain Themes in the Work of W. B. Yeats.* Colin Smythe, 1986.

Ryan, Meda. *Biddy Early: The Wise Woman of Clare.* Cork: Mercier P, 1978.

Sontag, Susan. *Illness as Metaphor.* Farrar, Straus and Giroux, 1978.

Úa Cadhain, Liam. *Venerable Archdeacon Cavanagh: Pastor of Knock Shrine, 1867-1897.* Knock Shrine Society, 2012.

Vendler, Helen. *Our Secret Discipline: Yeats and Lyric Form.* Harvard UP, 2007.

Wade, Allan. *A Bibliography of the Writings of W. B. Yeats.* Revised and edited by Russell K. Alspach. Rupert Hart-Davis, 1968.

Welch, Robert Anthony. *The Cold of May Day Monday: An Approach to Irish Literary History.* Oxford UP, 2014.

VIII. Book Chapters

McAuliffe, John. "Against Irish Studies: Reading Austin Clarke and His Critics." *New Voices in Irish Criticism*, edited by Patrick J. Matthews, vol. 1, Four Courts P, 2000, pp. 255–259.

McCormack, W. J. "Austin Clarke: The Poet as Scapegoat of Modernism." *Modernism and Ireland: The Poetry of the 1930s*, edited by Patricia Coughlan and Alex Davis, Cork UP, 1995, pp. 75–102.

O'Connor, Laura. "W. B. Yeats and Modernist Poetry." *The Cambridge Companion to Irish Modernism*, edited by Joe Cleary, Cambridge UP, 2014, pp. 77–94.

O'Donoghue, Bernard. "The Aisling." *A Companion to Poetic Genre*, edited by Erik Martiny, Blackwell, 2011, pp. 420–434.

Pethica, James. "'Our Kathleen': Yeats's Collaboration with Lady Gregory in the Writing of *Cathleen ni Houlihan*." *Yeats and Women*, edited by Deirdre Toomey, Macmillan, 1997, pp. 205–222.

———. "Patronage and Creative Exchange: Yeats, Lady Gregory and the Economy of Indebtedness." *Yeats and Women*, edited by Deirdre Toomey, Macmillan, 1997, pp. 168–204.

IX. Dissertations and Theses

Bell, Caehlin O'Malley. *Being Ireland: Lady Gregory in Cathleen Ni Houlihan*. 2008. Ohio State U, Master's dissertation. *OhioLINK*, rave.ohiolink.edu/etdc/view?acc_num=osu1211912530.

Pilz, Anna. *'The Return to the People': Empire, Class, and Religion in Lady Gregory's Dramatic Works*. 2013. U of Liverpool, PhD dissertation. *U of L Repository*, https://doi.org/10.17638/00014315.

X. Essays

Morris, William. *The Aims of Art*. Office of "The Commonweal," 1887.

O'Grady, Standish James. *Early Bardic Literature, Ireland*. Sampson Low, Searle, Marston, & Rivington / E. Ponsonby, 1879.

Pound, Ezra. *Make It New: Essays*. Faber and Faber, 1934.

Yeats, William Butler. *Essays and Introductions*. Macmillan, 1961.

XI. Interviews

Hynes, Garry. "In Conversation with Garry Hynes." Interview by Anna Pilz. *Irish Women's Writing (1880-1920) Network: Collaborations and Networks Symposium*, 3 Sept. 2021, irishwomenswritingnetwork.com/collaborations-and-networks-symposium/. Interview.

XII. Journal Articles

Alspach, Russell K. "Some Sources of Yeats's *The Wanderings of Oisin*." *Modern Language Association*, vol. 58, no. 3, 1943, pp. 849–66. *JSTOR*, https://doi.org/10.2307/458836.

Andrews, June. "'Wandering' and dementia." *British Journal of Community Nursing*, vol. 22, no. 7, 2017, pp. 322–23.

Ayres, Peter. "Wound dressing in World War I—The kindly *Sphagnum* Moss." *Field Bryology*, vol. 110, 2013, pp. 27–34.

Carlin, Aisling. "To 'make others see my dream as I had seen it': Yeats's aesthetics in *Cathleen ni Houlihan*." *Yeats Annual*, no. 19, 2013, pp. 65–76. *JSTOR*, https://doi.org/10.11647/OBP.0038.03.

Chaudhuri, Nani Gopal. "Some of the Results of the Great Bengal and Bihar Famine of 1770." *Proceedings of the Indian History Congress*, vol. 12, 1949, pp. 239–44. *JSTOR*, www.jstor.org/stable/44140542.

Correll, Timothy Corrigan. "Believers, Sceptics, and Charlatans: Evidential Rhetoric, the Fairies, and Fairy Healers in Irish Oral Narrative and Belief." *Folklore*, vol. 116, no. 1, 2005, pp. 1–18. *ProQuest*, https://doi.org/10.1080/0015587052000337680.

Foster, R. F. "Yeats and the Death of Lady Gregory." *Irish University Review*, vol. 34, no. 1, 2004, pp. 109–121. *JSTOR*, www.jstor.org/stable/25504960.

Gibson, Matthew. "Bram Stoker and the Treaty of Berlin (1878)." *Gothic Studies*, vol. 6, no. 2, 2004, pp. 236–51. *ProQuest*, https://doi.org/10.7227/GS.6.2.6.

Gilleard, Chris. "The other Victorians: age, sickness, and poverty in 19th-century Ireland." *Ageing & Society*, vol. 36, no. 6, 2016, pp. 1157–84. *ProQuest*, https://doi.org/10.1017/S0144686X15000240.

Gould, Warwick. "Lips and Ships, Peers and Tears: *Lacrimae Rerum* and Tragic Joy." *Yeats Annual*, no. 18, 2013, pp. 15–56. *JSTOR*, https://doi.org/10.11647/OBP.0028.03.

Hassett, Joseph M. "What Raftery Built." *Yeats Annual*, no. 18, 2013, pp. 97–106. *JSTOR*, https://doi.org/10.11647/OBP.0028.06.

Hickey, Raymond. "Salient features of Irish syntax." *Lingua Posnaniensis*, vol. 26, 1985, pp. 15–26.

Jenkins, Richard. "The Transformation of Biddy Early: From Local Reports of Magical Healing to Globalised New Age Fantasies." *Folklore*, vol. 118, no. 2, 2007, pp. 162–82. *JSTOR*, https://doi.org/10.1080/00155870701337379.

Kiernan, Thomas Joseph. "Lady Gregory and W. B. Yeats." *Dalhousie Review*, vol. 38, no. 3, 1958, pp. 295–306, hdl.handle.net/10222/58789.

Mattar, Sinéad Garrigan. "'Wage for Each People Her Hand Has Destroyed': Lady Gregory's Colonial Nationalism." *Irish University Review*, vol. 34, no. 1, 2004, pp. 49–66. *JSTOR*, www.jstor.org/stable/25504956.

McLean, Stuart. "Bodies from the Bog: Metamorphosis, Non-Human Agency and the Making of 'Collective' Memory." *TRAMES—Journal of the Humanities and Social Sciences*, vol. 12, no. 3, 2018, pp. 299–308.

Moses, Michael Valdez. "The Irish Vampire: *Dracula*, Parnell, and the Troubled Dreams of Nationhood." *Journal X: Journal in Culture and Criticism*, vol. 2, no. 1, 1997, pp. 66–112.

Murphy, Gerard. "Notes on *Cath Maige Tuired*." *Éigse: Journal of Irish Studies*, vol. 7, nos. 1–4, 1953–1955, pp. 191–98.

Nic Dhonnchadha, Aoibheann. "Medical writing in Irish." *Irish Journal of Medical Science*, vol. 169, no. 3, 2000, pp. 217–220.

Ó Conchubhair, Seán M. "The Congested Districts Board." *Irish Monthly*, vol. 69, no. 820, 1941, pp. 477–88. *JSTOR*, www.jstor.org/stable/20514937.

O'Conor, Norreys J. "Ireland's Literary Revival and Regional Writing." *Georgia Review*, vol. 1, no. 4, 1947, pp. 420–26. *JSTOR*, www.jstor.org/stable/41397564.

Ó Gráda, Cormac. "Revisiting the Bengal Famine of 1943–4." *History Ireland*, vol. 18, no. 4, 2010, pp. 36–39. *JSTOR*, www.jstor.org/stable/27823027.

Pethica, James. "'Uttering, Mastering it'? Yeats's Tower, Lady Gregory's Ballylee, and the Eviction of 1888." *Yeats Annual*, no. 21, 2018, pp. 213–268. *JSTOR*, https://doi.org/10.11647/OBP.0135.06.

Pilz, Anna. "Lady Gregory's 'Tree Planting.'" *Irish Forestry: Journal of the Society of Irish Foresters*, vol. 76, nos. 1 & 2, 2019, pp. 84–91, journal.societyofirishforesters.ie/index.php/forestry.

Purcell, Siobhán. "Beckett and Disability Biopolitics: The Case of Cuchulain." *Estudios Irlandeses*, vol. 14, no. 2, 2019, pp. 52–64. *Estudios Irlandeses*, https://doi.org/10.24162/EI2019-9171.

Quirici, Marion. "*Cathleen ni Houlihan and the Disability Aesthetics of Irish National Culture*." *Éire-Ireland*, vol. 50, nos. 3 & 4, 2015, pp. 74–93. Project MUSE, https://doi.org/10.1353/eir.2015.0017.

Rainsford, John. "Biddy Early's Limerick Connections." *Old Limerick Journal*, vol. 46, 2012, pp. 45–49. *Limerick City and County Council*, www.limerickcity.ie/Library/LocalStudies/BooksJournals/TheOldLimerickJournal/.

Schuchard, Ronald. "Yeats and Spirituality." *Princeton University Library Chronicle*, vol. 59, no. 3, 1998, pp. 321–49. *JSTOR*, www.jstor.org/stable/26509287.

Sidnell, Michael John. "The Allegory of Yeats's 'The Wanderings of Oisin.'" *Colby Library Quarterly*, vol. 15, no. 2, 1979, pp. 137–51, digitalcommons.colby.edu/cq/vol15/iss2/7/.

Stewart, Bruce. "Bram Stoker's Dracula: Possessed by the Spirit of the Nation?" *Irish University Review*, vol. 29, no. 2, 1999, pp. 238–55. *JSTOR*, www.jstor.org/stable/25484813.

Sullivan, Hannah. "How Yeats Learned to Scan." *Yeats Annual*, no. 21, 2018, pp. 3–38. *JSTOR*, www.jstor.org/stable/j.ctv8j415.9.

Whitaker, Thomas R. "The Early Yeats and the Pattern of History." *Modern Language Association*, vol. 75, no. 3, 1960, pp. 320–28. *JSTOR*, https://doi.org/10.2307/460343.

Whitehead, Lee M. "The Honey-Bees of W. B. Yeats' 'The Stare's Nest at My Window': Echoes of Orpheus." *Canadian Journal of Irish Studies*, vol. 5, no. 2, 1979, pp. 55–59. *JSTOR*, https://doi.org/10.2307/25512474.

XIII. Newspaper Articles

Burke, R. "The Last of the Irish Witches." *Weekly Irish Times (1876-1920)*. 10 Oct. 1903, p. 3, www.proquest.com/docview/850588121.

"House Burning." *Limerick Chronicle*. 28 Sept. 1853, www.limerickleader.ie/news/home/306356/limerick-chronicle-files-fact-fiction-fantasy-and-folklore-surrounding-biddy-early.html.

XIV. Online Articles and Book Reviews

Butler, Leah. "Biddy Early: The Wise Women of the West." *Women's Museum of Ireland*, 2013, www.womensmuseumofireland.ie/exhibits/biddy-early.

Cook, Daphnee, et al. "Madagascar: 'We Pretend to Cook Rice with Soil and Sand, Stones as Meat.'" *Save the Children*, 16 Nov. 2021, www.savethechildren.net/news/madagascar-%E2%80%9Cwe-pretend-cook-rice-soil-and-sand-stones-meat%E2%80%9D.

Geary, Lawrence. "Deadly disease: how the Great Famine led to outbreaks of illness." *RTÉ*. 29 Nov. 2020, www.rte.ie/history/the-great-irish-famine/2020/0721/1154625-deadly-disease-how-the-great-famine-led-to-outbreaks-of-illness/.

———. "Epidemic Diseases of the Great Famine." *History Ireland*, vol. 4, no. 1, 1996, www.historyireland.com/epidemic-diseases-of-the-great-famine/.

Hassett, Joseph M. "Escaping Lockdown with W. B. Yeats." *Dublin Review of Books*, 21 May 2020, drb.ie/escaping-lockdown-with-wb-yeats/.

"New Antimicrobial Streptomyces Species Discovered in Ancient Irish Soil." *Genetic Engineering and Biotechnology News*, 15 Jan. 2021, www.genengnews.com/news/new-antimicrobial-streptomyces-species-discovered-in-ancient-irish-soil/. Accessed 27 Apr. 2021.

Rainsford, John. “Feakle’s Biddy Early: a victim of ‘moral panic’?” *History Ireland*, vol. 20, no. 1, 2012, www.historyireland.com/feakles-biddy-early-a-victim-of-moral-panic/.

Sparks, Dana and Mayo Clinic Staff. “Alzheimer’s and dementia: Understand wandering and how to address it.” *Mayo Clinic*, 30 Nov. 2020, newsnetwork.mayoclinic.org/discussion/alzheimers-and-dementia-understand-wandering-and-how-to-address-it/. Accessed 20 Apr. 2021.

XV. Lectures and Debates

Foster, R. F. “Protestant Magic: W. B. Yeats and the Spell of Irish History.” Chatterton Lecture on Poetry. *Proceedings of the British Academy*, 5. Dec. 1989, British Academy, London.

Hansard, UK Parliament. “Purchase of Land and Congested Districts (Ireland) Bill.” *Hansard, Parliamentary Debates*, vol. 342, third series, 24 Mar. 1890, pars. 1696–1723, api.parliament.uk/historic-hansard/commons/1890/mar/24/purchase-of-land-and-congested- districts#column_1697.

Heaney, Seamus. “Crediting Poetry.” Nobel Lecture. The Nobel Prize in Literature, 7 Dec. 1995, Stockholm Concert Hall, Stockholm, www.nobelprize.org/prizes/literature/1995/heaney/lecture/.

XVI. Dictionaries, and Dictionary and Encyclopædia Definitions

“Congested, *Adj.* (1), (2a), and (2c).” *Oxford English Dictionary*, Oxford UP, 2023, www-oed-com.ucc.idm.oclc.org/view/Entry/39086.

“Cresset, *N.* (1a), (1b), and (C2).” *Oxford English Dictionary.* Oxford UP, 2023, www-oed-com.ucc.idm.oclc.org/view/Entry/44285.

Dictionary of Irish Biography. Dictionary of Irish Biography, 2023, www.dib.ie.

“East India Company.” *Encyclopædia Britannica*, 1 Dec. 2022, www.britannica.com/topic/East-India-Company.

“Hedonism, *N.*” *Oxford English Dictionary*, Oxford UP, 2023, www-oed-com.ucc.idm.oclc.org/view/Entry/85405.

Kiberd, Declan. “Synge, (Edmund) John Millington.” *Dictionary of Irish Biography*, Oct. 2009, https://doi.org/10.3318/dib.008429.v1.

“Lung Congestion.” *Encyclopædia Britannica*, 4 Apr. 2016, www.britannica.com/science/lung-congestion.

Martin, Elizabeth A. *Concise Medical Dictionary.* Oxford UP, 2010.

“Miasma, *N.* (1).” *Oxford English Dictionary*, Oxford UP, 2023, www-oed-com.ucc.idm.oclc.org/view/Entry/117825.

"Milky, *Adj.* (2b) and (4a)." *Oxford English Dictionary*, Oxford UP, 2023, www-oed-com.ucc.idm.oclc.org/view/Entry/118467.
"Moss, *N.*1 (7)." *Oxford English Dictionary*, Oxford UP, 2023, www-oed-com.ucc.idm.oclc.org/view/Entry/122565.
"Overhang, *N.* (1b) and *V.* (1b)." *Oxford English Dictionary*, Oxford UP, 2023, www-oed-com.ucc.idm.oclc.org/view/Entry/134666; www-oed-com.ucc.idm.oclc.org/view/Entry/134667.
"Pishogue, *N.* (1)." *Oxford English Dictionary*, Oxford UP, 2023, www-oed-com.ucc.idm.oclc.org/view/Entry/144582.
"Resuscitation, *N.* (2a)." *Oxford English Dictionary*, Oxford UP, 2023, www-oed-com.ucc.idm.oclc.org/view/Entry/164123.
"Revival, *N.* (1a) and (2c)." *Oxford English Dictionary*, Oxford UP, 2023, www-oed-com.ucc.idm.oclc.org/view/Entry/164908.
"Tuatha Dé Danann." *Encyclopædia Britannica*, 27 Jan. 2023, www.britannica.com/topic/Tuatha-De-Danann.
"Wandering, *Adj.* (2g) and *N.* (1a)." *The Oxford English Dictionary*, Oxford UP, 2023, www-oed-com.ucc.idm.oclc.org/view/Entry/225442; www-oed-com.ucc.idm.oclc.org/view/Entry/225441.
"Wander, *V.* (2e)." *Oxford English Dictionary*, Oxford UP, 2023, www-oed-com.ucc.idm.oclc.org/view/Entry/225437.
"Weir, *N.* (1a)." *Oxford English Dictionary*. Oxford UP, 2023, www-oed-com.ucc.idm.oclc.org/view/Entry/226913.
"Well-being, *N.*" *Oxford English Dictionary*, Oxford UP, 2023, www-oed-com.ucc.idm.oclc.org/view/Entry/227050.
"Well, *N.*1 (1b) and *N.*2 (1a)." *Oxford English Dictionary*, Oxford UP, 2023, www-oed-com.ucc.idm.oclc.org/view/Entry/226978; www-oed-com.ucc.idm.oclc.org/view/Entry/226979.

XVII. Manuscripts and Archive Materials

Cath Maige Tuired: The Second Battle of Mag Tuired. Circa. 1501–1600, British Library, London, Harleian MS 5280, fols. 63a-70b. Manuscript.
Duffy, Charles Gavan. *The Ballad Poetry of Ireland.* 1874, National Library of Ireland, Dublin, MS 40,568/77. Manuscript.
Reynolds, Horace M. *Horace Mason Reynolds's Papers.* 8 July 1927, Harvard Library, Harvard, b Ms Am 1787 [5803]. Manuscript.
Yeats, Lily. *Copies, with annotations, made by Lily Yeats, of seven letters of John Butler Yeats to Susan Yeats, of Sligo, 1872-3.* 1872–1873, National Library of Ireland, Dublin, MS 2064. Manuscript.

XVIII. Photographs and Images

Image of *The Well of All-Healing*. 1897, John J. Burns Library, Boston College.

XIX. Websites, Webpages, Databases, Online Tools, and Online Documents

"Collaborations and Networks Symposium 2021." *Irish Women's Writing (1880-1920) Network*, 2021, irishwomenswritingnetwork.com/virtualsymposium. Accessed 8 Jan. 2022.

Coole Park Nature Reserve. Coole Park Nature Reserve, 2023, www.coolepark.ie. Accessed 20 Oct. 2021.

Druid Theatre. Druid Performing Arts, 2023, www.druid.ie. Accessed 1 Oct. 2021.

"The Main Manuscript Collection." *National Folklore Collection*, 2023, www.duchas.ie/en/cbe. Accessed 6 May 2023.

"Nature & Wildlife." *Coole Park Nature Reserve*, 2023, www.coolepark.ie/nature-wildlife/. Accessed 20 Oct. 2021.

New York Public Library. "'A Friend's Illness': William Butler Yeats (1865–1939)." *New York Public Library*, 2023, www.nypl.org/events/exhibitions/2910/galleries/2914/item/3521. Accessed 22 Apr. 2021.

———. "Lady Gregory as Cathleen ni Houlihan." *New York Public Library*, 2023, www.nypl.org/events/exhibitions/galleries/section-7-they-came-swallows/item/3578. Accessed 15 Jan. 2022.

———. "Playing Cathleen ni Houlihan." *New York Public Library*, 2023, www.nypl.org/events/exhibitions/galleries/section-7-they-came-swallows/item/3595. Accessed 15 Jan. 2022.

Orwant, Jon and William Brockman. *Google Books Ngram Viewer*. Google, Dec. 2010, books.google.com/ngrams. Accessed 22 Apr. 2021.

"Poets and Dreamers: Studies and Translations from the Irish." *National Library of Ireland*, 2023, catalogue.nli.ie/Record/vtls000071494. Accessed 4 Dec. 2021.

"Regions of Ireland." *Discovering Ireland Vacations*, 2023, www.discoveringireland.com/regions-of-ireland/. Accessed 18 Oct. 2022.

Rubel, William. "History of the Stone Soup Folktale from 1720 to Now." *StoneSoup*, 2023, stonesoup.com/about-the-childrens-art-foundation-and-stone-soup-magazine/history-of-the-stone-soup-story-from-1720-to-now/. Accessed 11 Jan. 2022.

"The Schools' Collection." *National Folklore Collection*, 2023, www.duchas.ie/en/cbes. Accessed 6 May 2023.

"Visions and Beliefs in the West of Ireland." *National Library of Ireland*, 2023, catalogue.nli.ie/Record/vtls000142820. Accessed 10 Mar. 2023.

"Wandering." *Google Books Ngram Viewer: 1800-2019: English Fiction 2019*, Jon Orwant and William Brockman, Google, Dec. 2010, books.google.com/ngrams/graph?content=wandering&year_start=1800&year_end=2019&corpus=en-fiction-2019&smoothing=3.

"Well-being." *Google Books Ngram Viewer: 1900-2019: English Fiction 2019*. Jon Orwant and William Brockman. Google, Dec. 2010, books.google.com/ngrams/graph?content=well-being&year_start=1800&year_end=2019&corpus=en-fiction-2019&smoothing=3. Accessed 17 Oct. 2022.

Index[1]

A
Abbey Theatre, 6n4, 21n5, 22n8, 95, 95n12, 104, 134–137, 180–183, 197n2
Ability, 40, 75, 94n6, 132, 177–180, 196
AE (George William Russell), 64–68, 170
  "Well of All-Healing, The," 64, 65, 170
Aesthetic, 28n20, 64, 105n25, 188, 197
Aestheticist, 28n20, 64
Aetiology, 20, 36, 68
Ag fánaíocht, 26
Aghamore, County Mayo, 176n2
Agriculture, 161
Ailment, 13, 35, 48, 49, 72–75, 86, 114, 122, 153, 172
Aisling, 105–107, 105n25
Anapestic feet, 36
Anapestic hexameter, 28, 35, 53
Anaphora, 40, 42, 112
Anthropology, 3
Anti-colonial, 95, 97
Anti-colonialism, 106
Anti-health, 193, 196
Anti-imperial, 93, 115
Anti-imperialist, 93, 115
Anti-Revival, 196
Anti-self, 179, 187
Antrim, County, 181
Apples, 31, 74, 114, 155
Aran Islands, 95, 161–163, 171, 177–179, 182
Archetype, 107
Artist-healer, 128, 148
Athair-talav, 129, 133, 136–138, 140–142
Athenry, County Galway, 184
Avant-garde drama, 25, 187
Axiom, 94

[1] Note: Page numbers followed by 'n' refer to notes.

H. M. Walker-Dunseith, *Traditional Medicine in the Irish Literary Revival*, New Directions in Irish and Irish American Literature,
https://doi.org/10.1007/978-3-031-82459-3

B
Ballyhaunis, County Mayo, 176n2
Ballylee, 53, 54, 58–79, 86–87, 98, 122–123, 170, 194
Banshee, 108
Bardic poetry, 106
Bean chaointe, 92, 109
Bean feasa, 92, 108–109, 126, 195
Bean ghlúine, 92, 109, 126, 195
  See also Midwife
Bean sí, 108
  See also Banshee
Beehive, 176, 176n1
Beekeeping, 80–82, 80n29
Bees, 57, 60, 61, 77–87
Beggars, 102, 118, 128, 142, 151, 186
Bengal Famine, 96
Big House, 96
  See also Coole House, County Galway
Blake, William, 42, 43, 52
Blind, 12–13, 18, 20–24, 29–32, 35, 36, 82, 83, 120, 149–150, 160–164, 166–173, 180–186, 188–192
Blindness, 12–13, 82, 83, 160, 166–172, 180–186, 190–192
Blunt, Anne, 97–98
Blunt, Wilfrid Scawen, 93–98, 122, 134
Body, 2–9, 12, 20, 21, 23, 27–33, 35–39, 45–54, 64n7, 68n10, 68n11, 75, 75n17, 75n18, 82n36, 116–118, 140–145, 153, 155–156, 188, 194, 196, 197
Bog bodies, 75, 75n18
Botanist, 46, 121, 124
Bridges, Robert, 28, 28n21

C
Cailleach, 9–10, 92, 92n1, 103, 106–110, 118, 126, 195
Campbell, Joseph, 101, 107
Capitalist, 13, 193, 197
Carlyle, Thomas, 94
Cath Maige Tuired, 34, 34n24, 34n25, 35, 43, 185
Catholicism, 69–71, 94, 95, 173
Cavanagh, Venerable Archdeacon, 173n15
Ceathair Aluinn, 178
  See also Four Beautiful Persons, The
Celtic Christmas, A, 65, 170
Celtic Theatre, 95
Celtic Twilight, 18, 74
Choctaw tribe, 144
Christianity, 26n16, 31, 151
Clare, County, 26, 63–64, 68–70, 71n13, 72n14, 75, 108, 114, 120–124, 131–133, 185
Clarke, Austin, 101
Clontarf, Battle of, 75
Coimín, Dáithí, 26n17
Coimín, Micheál, 26, 26n16, 26n17, 66n8
Colonial, 94–102, 106, 114, 120, 126, 147, 171, 195, 196
Colonialism, 10, 96, 101, 106, 120, 126, 195
Colonisation, 62
Congested Districts Board (CDB), 12, 161–171, 192
Congestion, 12, 160–166, 197
Connemara, County Mayo, 10, 86, 121, 160–164, 171, 183, 188, 197
Convalescence, 1, 53
Conventional medicine, 6, 44
Coole, County Galway, 9, 21n5, 23n10, 54, 58–63, 67–69, 74–84, 86, 93–96, 93n5, 98, 108, 115, 121–124, 126, 148, 184, 194
Coole House, County Galway, 23n10, 96
Coole Park, County Galway, 9, 58–63, 68, 80, 92–96, 124n37, 131, 148

Corbière, Tristram, 100
Cork, 68, 131
Cough cure, 10, 93, 123
Country of the Young, 113, 128
Countryside, 3–10, 25, 62, 107, 114–116, 131, 141–147, 163, 189, 198
See also Irish countryside
Culpeper, Nicholas, 45n30, 46
Cultural nationalism, 106, 197n2
Cures, 3–8, 12, 29–35, 43–49, 67, 71n13, 72–79, 72n14, 82, 83, 86, 87, 99, 113n31, 114–117, 120–124, 126, 139–140n10, 152–156, 173n15, 176–178, 182–187, 194, 195, 198
Curing water, 186

D
Decongestion, 12, 162, 166
De Danaan, 18, 25, 30, 33–35, 42, 48, 49
Dew, 29, 35, 39, 74–75, 80
Diet, 4–6, 75n17, 95
Disability, 186, 195, 196
Disease, 5, 20, 34, 61–62, 63n5, 68n10, 72n14, 81, 94, 94n6, 96, 117, 122, 185n10
Doctor, 6, 28, 44, 47, 48, 62n4, 63n5, 76, 92, 99, 112–125, 131–133, 138, 141, 152–155, 183
Dome, The, 28n20, 64
Donegal, County, 125
Doppelgänger, 105
Down, County, 181
Druid Theatre, 92, 134
Dublin, County, 4, 11, 21n5, 23n10, 43, 50, 86, 95, 99–102, 105, 128, 179, 181, 194
Duffy, Charles Gavan, 33

E
Early, Biddy, 9–12, 62–79, 87, 108–110, 114, 121–123, 126, 130–132, 194–196
Easter Rising, 8, 58, 84, 103n23
East India Company, 95, 96
Elixir of life, 36, 113, 152
Emigration, 5, 12, 162–164
Ennis, County Clare, 71
Ethnography, 171
Eucharistic and Marian Apparition, 173
Evelyn, John, 4, 119, 123–124
Silva, 4, 119, 123–124
Eyesight, 3, 9–12, 86, 121, 123n36, 134, 160–164, 174, 182–185, 190, 196

F
Fagan, 10, 86, 121
See also Kirwan
Fairies, 7, 10, 18, 18n2, 32, 40, 45n30, 49, 63, 69, 71–77, 86, 108n28, 121–125, 132, 133, 142
Famine pot, 144–146
Feakle, County Clare, 70, 74n16, 120
Fearavan, 129, 133, 136, 137, 140–142
Fenian, 19, 23, 26, 30–32, 50, 53, 117–118, 172, 185
Fianna, 118
Fir Bolgs, 185
First World War, 8, 58, 75, 84
Flannel, 93–94, 99, 109, 121
Flowers, 8, 25, 28, 29, 33–35, 43, 45–47, 50, 60, 178
Folk healer, 6–10, 63, 92, 122, 126, 195
Folklore-collecting practice, 66n9, 67, 102
Folklore collection, 2, 9–11, 46, 48, 59, 70, 114, 128, 139, 155–156, 176n2

Folk medical practices, 99
Folk stories, 95, 120, 152n13
Folk tradition, 106
Fomorians, 185
Forester's panacea, 4, 10, 123–124, 126, 196
Forgetfulness, 19–24, 28–32, 97–98
Foster, John Wilson, 1, 21n5, 22, 22n9, 23n10, 24n11, 51, 51n37, 62n4, 73, 73n15, 111, 121
  Apprentice Mage, The, 21n5, 22n9, 24n11, 51, 51n37, 73, 73n15, 121
  Arch-Poet, The, 51, 62n4
Four Beautiful Persons, The, 178, 182
  See also Ceathair Aluinn
Free verse, 28, 28n22, 29
Fresh air, 67

G

Galway Bay, 95, 171
Galway, County, 63n6, 72n14, 75–77, 82n36, 95, 95n10, 100, 112, 131–133, 139n10, 160, 171, 178
Germ theory, 68
Gonne, Maud, 21, 22, 22n9, 60, 60n3, 102
Gort, County Galway, 63n6, 70, 77–78, 131–132
Gregory, Augusta
  "Blessed Patrick of the Bells," 185
  Book of Saints and Wonders, 185
  "Brigit, The Mary of the Gael," 185n10
  Coole, autobiography, 3, 123, 124
  Cuchulain of Muirthemne, 96, 99, 100, 110, 113n31, 153
  Diaries, 98, 143, 144, 151n12
  "Felons of Our Land, The," 104
  Gaol Gate, The, 93n4
  Gods and Fighting Men, 113, 117n33, 118, 155
  Golden Apple, The, 114, 116–118, 154–155
  "Great Wonders of the Olden Time," 185, 191
  "Herb-Healing," 10–12, 128–142
  "Herbs, Charms, and Wise Women," 10, 119, 128, 138, 139, 139n10, 141–142, 153
  "Hunt of Slieve Cuilinn, The," 118
  Journals, 102, 103n23, 124
  Kiltartan Poetry Book, The, 107, 113, 142, 184
  Marriage, The, 129, 148–150
  Poets and Dreamers, 10–12, 113n31, 128–156, 195
  Rising of the Moon, The, 93n4, 129, 148–151
  "Seers and Healers," 10, 70, 72, 86, 120–122
  Seventy Years, 93–94, 120, 122
  "Sons of Tuireann, The," 113, 117n33, 155
  Travelling Man, The, 129, 150, 151n12
  Visions and Beliefs, 10–12, 63n5, 70–74, 71n13, 72n14, 116, 120–124, 128–133, 135–142, 155–156, 195
Gregory, Robert, 21n5, 93, 96, 98, 128
Gregory, William Henry, 92, 95, 110, 123
Griffith, Arthur Joseph, 181
Gross Domestic Product (GDP), 164
Guise, 9, 92, 106, 110
Gwynn, Stephen, 104

H

"Hag of Beare, The," 106, 107
Happiness, 12, 80, 94–95, 98, 132, 161, 164, 169, 179

Healing moss, 9, 72–73, 77, 79, 87, 122, 194
Healing properties, 35, 47, 53, 79, 86, 99
Healing well, 13, 176–179, 184–185, 187–193, 196
Healthcare, 6, 44
Heaney, Seamus, 41, 75n18, 80, 80n28
Hedonism, 161n6
Hellebore, 3, 45, 45n30, 46
Herbalism, 3, 12, 123, 135, 138, 156, 195
Herbalist, 10, 46, 125, 129, 135
See also Irish herbalist
Herbal medicine, 34, 43, 45, 72n14, 119, 129, 152, 193, 195, 196
Hibernia, 114
Hiberno-English, 100, 165
Hogan, Michael, 71
Holistic care, 7
Holly, 113
Holy water, 166, 181, 186
Holy well, 12, 172, 176, 178, 182
Homogeneity, 165
Homogenous, 13, 162
Homonym, 12, 13, 160, 191, 197
Honey, 29, 45, 74–76, 79–87, 114, 124
Honeybees, 77, 79–80, 84, 84n37, 86
Hot stones, 116–118, 155
Hunger, 5, 69, 96, 122, 130, 145–147, 149–152, 181n7
Hyde, Douglas, 4, 95n11, 129n2, 147

I
Iambic pentameter, 29, 35
Iambic tetrameter, 31, 52
Ibsen, Henrik, 41, 106, 116
Ibsenite naturalism, 116
Idealism, 116, 148
Ill health, 9, 58–59, 66n9, 169–170, 179, 180
Imagery, 26n16, 84, 98, 98n15
Indigenous, 8, 54, 95, 194
Industrialisation, 38, 39
Industrialism, 38
Industrial Revolution, 38
Inisheer, County Galway, 95
Inishmore, 12, 162, 171, 176, 178, 182, 198
Irish ballad, 67
Irish bards, 29
Irish Civil War, 83, 85
Irish country life, 69
Irish countryside, 8–10, 62, 114–116, 141–147, 198
Irish culture, 18, 181
Irish dialogue poetry, 26n16
Irish districts, 12, 166
Irish doctors, 6n3
Irish Dramatic Movement, 85–86, 85n39, 187
Irish epics, 96n14
Irish Famine, 4–6, 43, 44, 70, 144–146, 188
Irish folklore, 8, 54, 75, 87, 99, 102, 194
Irish folk medicine, 7, 75n17, 82, 86
Irish Free State, 2, 24n13, 58n1, 196
Irish healing practices, 7, 12
Irish herbalist, 129
Irish heritage, 8, 35, 36, 50, 53, 54, 58, 79n26
Irish history, 58n1, 111n29
Irish identity, 3, 147
Irish independence, 104, 150
Irish language, 4–6, 9, 26, 35, 50–54, 58–61, 86, 95, 101, 106–108, 120–121, 133, 147, 183, 194
Irish legend, 10, 41, 135
Irish life, 1, 3, 4, 13, 184, 188, 191, 196
Irish Literary Revival, 1, 8, 24n13, 58, 101, 125, 180
Irish Literary Theatre, 95n12

Irish literature, 2, 26, 29, 53, 92n1, 104, 106–111, 119, 195, 196
Irish lore, 82
Irish lyrical poem, 26n17
Irish medical humanities, 2
Irish moss, 75n17
Irish mythology, 31, 49, 106, 119, 173, 185
Irish narratives, 95
Irish nationalism, 39
Irish National Theatre Society, 95n12
Irishness, 196
Irish novelist, 95n9, 101
Irish Ossianic poetry, 27n19
Irish past, 19, 36, 49, 62
Irish people, 21, 84, 106, 112, 142, 144, 162, 168, 191
Irish poet, 33, 80, 101, 145
Irish remedies, 6, 117
Irish Renaissance, 43, 95n10, 103
Irish Revival, 1–2, 4–8, 11–13, 24, 25, 43, 54, 87, 110, 116, 156, 171, 177, 180, 186, 190–192, 194, 195, 197
Irish Sea, 181
Irish society, 6, 20, 131n3, 163
Irish soil, 7, 25
Irish superstition, 32
Irish traditions, 87, 106, 131
Irish verse, 67
Irony, 12, 39, 43, 94, 112, 130, 146, 163, 173–174, 177, 178, 197

J
Japanese Noh drama, 187
Joyce, James, 4, 97
  Dubliners, 4
  Ulysses, 97
Juniper, 124–126, 196
Juniperus communis, 124–125

K
Keats, John, 40, 179
Keener, 108, 109
Keening-woman, 92, 109
Kildare, County, 181n8
Killala, County Mayo, 103
Killeenan, County Clare, 149–150
Kiltartan, 11, 63, 100–101, 107, 112–114, 134, 139, 142, 184–186, 195
Kiltartan dialect, 139
Kiltartanese, 100–101
Kiltartan parish, County Galway, 99, 112
Kirwan, 121
  See also Fagan
Knock, County Mayo, 12, 173–174, 176n2

L
Lalor, James Fintan, 111
Land League, 111
Land of the Young, 8, 54, 194
Land War, 111
Laois, County, 181n8
Legend, 1–4, 10, 18, 19, 29, 32, 33, 39, 41, 71n12, 75, 76n19, 82, 102, 106–107, 109, 117–118, 131, 135, 184
Leinster, 191
Leisure, 39–43, 47
Leitrim, 82
Lifestyle, 10, 60n3, 126
Locus amoenus, 182
  See also Pleasant place
Logan, Patrick, 6–7, 75n17, 82, 82n34, 82n35, 82n36, 99, 125, 176
  Making the Cure, 6, 75n17, 82, 99, 125
Longford, County, 152n14, 181n8
Louth, County, 181n8

M

Mac Cumhaill, Fionn, 30, 117
MacDonagh, Thomas, 109
Macpherson, James, 26, 27n19, 29
Madagascar Famine, 145
Madder dye, 94, 99
Malnutrition, 96
Martyn, Edward, 63, 95, 106
Materialism, 8, 11, 38, 40–42, 106, 116, 128, 130, 150
Mayo, 12, 20, 103, 122, 162n8, 165, 173, 176n2
Meath, County, 181n8
Medical humanities, 2–3
Medicinal herbs, 8, 25
Medicinal properties, 160
Memories/memory, 8, 11, 18–20, 23, 25, 28, 32, 33, 36, 37, 41, 49, 50, 70, 71, 108, 111–112, 126, 131, 132, 145, 169, 184, 187, 188, 195
Memory disorders, 8, 20
Merriman, Brian, 107
Metamorphosis, 36, 80n27, 103
Metaphor, 1, 2, 4, 12, 20–23, 30, 82, 102, 113, 116, 119, 133, 147, 165, 176, 193, 197n2, 198
Miasmas, 27, 67–68
Miasmatic hypothesis, 68
Middleton, Lucy, 49
Midwife, 92, 109, 126, 195
Migration, 162
Millboards, 9, 62, 64, 77, 79, 87, 194
Mill, John Stuart, 42
Millstream, 74, 76n19, 123
Millwheels, 9, 64, 68, 72–74, 122
Mitchell, Thomas Duché, 46
Modernisation, 163, 165, 171
Modernism, 1n1, 25, 25n14, 100, 101, 170, 177n3, 188, 194, 197
Modernity, 7, 9, 12–13, 61, 100, 162, 165, 171, 174, 192, 193, 196, 197
Modern medicine, 6–7, 20, 121
Monkshood, 44, 46
Monosyllabic tetrameter, 32
Montesquieu, 94, 94n7
Moore, George, 95n9, 101
Moore, T. Sturge, 53
Morality, 198
Morris, William, 38, 39
Moss, 8, 9, 25, 53, 63–64, 72–77, 79–84, 87, 122, 194
  See also Irish moss
Mystical, 8, 41, 42, 69, 87, 194
Myth, 3, 9, 62, 80, 108, 114, 125, 125n38, 196
Mythology, 10, 18n2, 31, 39, 48–50, 52, 52n39, 80n29, 81, 106, 108–109, 113, 114, 119, 125, 153–155, 172–173, 185

N

National Folklore Collection (NFC), 46, 114, 176n2
Nationalism, 4, 7, 39, 104, 106, 135, 197
  See also Irish nationalism
Naturalism, 106, 116, 187
Naturalist dramaturgy, 106
Nature, 7–8, 13, 18, 39, 41, 42, 53, 61, 75, 80, 85, 98, 117, 124n37, 147, 162, 170, 174, 177n3, 179, 180, 188, 196
Negative capability, 39, 40
New Poor Law, 5
Nic Shiubhlaigh, Máire, 102
  See also Walker, Mary
Nutrition, 4–6, 96

O
Offaly, County, 154n16, 181n8
Ó Flannghaile, Tomás, 26n17
O'Grady, Standish James, 13, 27n19, 29
 Early Bardic Literature, 13, 27n19, 29
Old age, 8, 19, 36, 118, 172
Old Irish cure, 75
O'Looney, Bryan, 26n17
O'Rahilly, Egan, 107
Oral Irish tradition, 131
Oral tradition, 107
Orientalism, 97, 98, 98n15
Ossianic, 27n19, 172
O'Sullivan, Seumas, 101
Oxygenation, 68

P
Paralysis, 4
Peasant plays, 187
Peasantry, 63n5, 71, 76, 76n19, 97, 102, 165, 170, 184, 197
Penal Laws, 5
Persse, Dudley, 94, 94n8, 101, 102
Persse, Frances, 115
Persse, Robert, 94
Pettigrew, Thomas Joseph, 45, 45n29, 46, 83
Philosophers' stone, 36n26, 75
Physician, 7–8, 33, 34, 34n25, 46, 48, 113n31, 121, 129, 151n11, 153, 185
Plantain, 44, 45n30, 47, 134
Pleasant place, 182
Post-Famine, 5
Pound, Ezra, 28n22, 100, 100n19, 111, 187
Pre-Raphaelite Brotherhood, 38
Preservation, 36, 37, 54, 75n17, 140–141, 176
Preventative care, 6n3
Primitivism, 6n4, 100, 165
Proselytism, 101
Protestantism, 95, 101–102, 111–112
Public health, 4–6

Q
Quinn, John, 63n6, 77, 77n22, 77n23

R
Raftery, Anthony, 121, 129, 148–150
Rationalism, 8, 38, 40–42
Realism, 106, 187
Regular verse, 28, 29
Rejuvenation, 11, 60n3, 92, 113–114, 119, 186, 195, 197
Remedies, 3–6, 10, 23, 35, 44, 48, 49, 75n17, 82, 82n36, 87, 99–101, 116–117, 120–121, 124, 131, 153–155, 162, 171, 176, 193, 194, 196
Restoration, 8–10, 13, 58–62, 67, 82, 110, 178
Resuscitation, 1, 13, 57
Revival, *see* Irish Revival
Revivalism, 181, 197
Revivalist, 3, 10, 37, 50, 61, 119, 122, 172, 177, 193
Reynolds, James, 131
Rheumatism, 46, 98–99
Romanticism, 25n14, 40, 41, 197
Roxborough, County Galway, 94, 100, 101
Ruane, Bridget, 10–12, 128–134, 140, 141, 154–156, 195, 196
Russell, George William (AE), 64, 170

S
Said, Edward W., 97, 98
St. Berchán, 176
St. Brendan of Birr, 176

St. Brigid's Cross, 154
St. Ciaran, 191
St. Conall, 176
St. Fursey, 176
St. Patrick, 18–20, 26n16, 29–32, 41, 172, 176n2, 185, 191, 193
St. Patrick's Well, 176n2
Salutary, 59, 67, 75, 87, 114, 183–184, 194
Schools' Manuscript Collection, The (NFCS), 46, 47, 72n14, 99, 114, 125, 131n3, 151–154, 176n2
Scientific, 2–3, 7, 69, 87, 194
Seanchaí, 3
The Second Battle of Mag Tuired, 34, 34n24, 34n25, 43, 185
Self-heal, 44, 46
Self-redefinition, 9, 92
Self-reinvention, 10, 92, 95, 98, 99, 120, 122
Shakespear, Olivia, 60, 63n6
Shawe-Taylor, Elizabeth, 101, 115
Sheepskin, 117, 155
Sickness, 5, 20, 61, 68, 74, 82–83, 114, 121–122, 149–153, 179–180, 183, 186
Sight, 3, 12, 49, 80n28, 86, 106, 121, 123n36, 134, 160, 163, 166–168, 172–174, 178, 182, 185–186, 190–191, 196
Slanlus, 46, 129, 133–134, 137–142
Sligo, County, 49, 67, 73, 178, 189
Sphagnum moss, 75
Standardisation, 163
Starvation, 4–6, 96, 181n7
Stephens, James, 4
Stoker, Bram, 111, 111n29
Storytelling, 3, 7, 119
  See also Seanchaí
Strength, 8–9, 13, 18, 19, 31, 33, 42, 47, 50, 54, 61, 64n7, 110, 112, 180, 184, 193, 194, 196
Symbol, 9–12, 20, 26, 28, 32, 41, 54, 58n1, 66n9, 79, 79n26, 84–85, 87, 106, 109, 116, 128, 145, 151, 154, 155, 195
Symbolic language, 10–12, 128, 155, 195
Symbolism, 26n16, 28, 87, 151
Symptom, 5n2, 8, 18, 20, 25, 32, 36, 113, 162, 197
Synge, John Millington
  Aran Islands, The, 162, 176–178
  Autobiography, 169, 180n6
  "Boat Builders, The," 171
  "From Galway to Gorumna," 160
  "From the Congested Districts," 197
  "In West Kerry," 160n3, 183
  In Wicklow, West Kerry and Connemara, 160n3, 164, 171, 183, 188, 197
  "Landlord's Garden in County Wicklow, A," 181
  "Oppression of the Hills, The," 164–165, 172, 197
  Playboy of the Western World, The, 169n11, 181
  "Possible Remedies," 171
  Well of the Saints, The, 12, 13, 160, 163, 166, 170, 172, 176–178, 180–181, 186–193, 196

T

Thoor Ballylee, 8–10, 53, 54, 58–67, 77–79, 86–87, 94n6, 98, 170n13, 194
Thoreau, Henry David, 189
Tír na nÓg, 8, 31, 32, 54, 110, 113–114, 194
Tobar an Ceathrar Álainn, 12, 176
Tobar Phádraig, 176n2
Tolstoy, Leo, 94n7

Tower, 8–10, 53, 64–67, 77–87, 194
Traditional Irish belief, 99
Traditional Irish medicine, 8, 25, 82, 155
Traditional Irish professions, 164
Traditional medicine, 1–4, 9–12, 20, 44, 112, 125, 132, 134, 140, 155, 193, 198
Tramp, 10, 69–70, 128–130, 133–146, 148–152, 156, 195
Transformation, 11, 95, 97, 105–106, 109, 122, 126, 149, 155, 195
Trimeter, 66
Trochaic heptamer, 75
Tuatha Dé Danann, 18n2, 185
Tulira, County Galway, 59, 60n3, 63
Tynan, Katharine, 50, 67

U
Ulster, 96, 142
Ulster Cycle, 96
Ungrateful city, 189
Urbs ingrata, 189
  See also Ungrateful city
Utilitarianism, 13, 39, 42, 110, 161n6, 193

V
Ventilation, 67
Vers libre, 28
Vervain, 3, 44–46, 45n30
Virgil, 80–82, 80n27
Vision poem, 106, 107

W
Walker, Mary, 102
Wandering, 8, 17–55, 169, 193, 194
Wavering, 18, 19n3, 21, 27, 52
Weakness, 8–9, 18, 19, 32, 42, 47, 54, 193, 194
Welfare, 121, 160
Well-being, 12, 23, 105, 109, 126, 160–162, 174, 195, 196
Wellness, 12, 160–162, 171, 191, 196, 198
Well of the Four Beauties, 167, 176, 182–183
Westmeath, County, 99, 181n8
Wexford, County, 181
Wicklow, County, 160n3, 164, 165, 166n10, 170–172, 181–183, 183n9, 188, 197
Wilde, Jane, 3–4, 13, 32–35, 44–48, 45n30, 75–79, 82–83, 86, 87, 108, 117, 184, 194
  Ancient Cures, 3–4, 32–35, 44, 47, 76, 76n20, 76n21, 79n26, 82, 86
  Ancient Legends, 3, 75, 76n19, 117–118, 184
  “Doctor’s Visit, The,” 76
  “Fenian Knights, The,” 117
  “Horned Women, The,” 75, 184
  Poems by Speranza, 108
Wise woman, 6, 10, 63–64, 72n14, 92, 108, 114, 126, 138, 141–142, 153, 195

Y
Yeats, Jane Grace, 73
Yeats, Michael, 77n23, 78n25
Yeats, Robert Corbet, 73
Yeats, Susan (Yeats’s mother), 73, 73n15
Yeats, Susan Mary (Lily; Yeats’s sister), 73n15
Yeats, William Butler
  “Acre of Grass, An,” 64n7

At the Hawk's Well, 119, 119n34, 186–190
Autobiographies, 20–22, 23n10, 36, 36n26, 49, 49n34, 50, 50n35, 59–60, 60n3, 67–68, 73n15, 85–87, 85n39, 85n40, 108, 189
"Blood and the Moon," 53, 57–58
Cat and the Moon, The, 185–186
Cathleen Ni Houlihan (with Augusta Gregory), 92–93, 102–110, 138, 148, 196
"Celtic Element in Literature, The," 41
Celtic Twilight, The, 9, 64, 84, 86, 125
Countess Cathleen, The, 3, 21, 22, 22n7, 22n8, 43–48, 54, 84, 84n37, 95n12, 191
"Down by the Salley Gardens," 67
Dramatis Personae, 23n10, 60, 68, 73n15
"Dust Hath Closed Helen's Eye," 64
Early Poems and Stories, 24
"Ephemera," 52, 52n39
Essays and Introductions, 28, 41, 92, 179
Estrangement, 20, 50
Fairy and Folk Tales, 76, 76n19, 184
Four Years, 36, 85n40, 189
"Friend's Illness, A," 21n5
"Hosting of the Sidhe, The," 108
Hour-Glass, The, 137–138
Ideas of Good and Evil, 28n20, 41n27
"In the Seven Woods," (poem), 80
In the Seven Woods (poetry collection), 60
"Ireland After Parnell," 85n40
Irish Dramatic Movement, The, 85n39, 86n41, 187
"Irish Witch Doctors," 121
King's Threshold, The, 148
"Lake of Innisfree, The," 84
"Lapis Lazuli," 80n27
Last Poems, 104
"Madness of King Goll, The," 52, 52n39
"Man and the Echo, The," 104
"Meditations in Time of Civil War," 62n4, 83
Memoirs, 60
Michael Robartes and the Dancer, 62n4, 77n23, 78n25
Mythologies, 9, 64, 72, 84, 87, 108–109, 125, 132
"People's Theatre, A," 187
Poems by W. B. Yeats, 18n1, 22, 24n12, 48, 49, 84
Pot of Broth, The (with Augusta Gregory), 10–12, 69–71, 128–129, 133–146, 148–152, 156, 195
"Queen and the Fool, The," 132
Reveries Over Childhood and Youth, 49, 50n35, 85n40, 108
Rose, The, 52
"Sailing to Byzantium," 53
"Second Coming, The," 194
"Shadowy Waters, The," 69
"Song of the Rosy Cross, The," 75
"Song of Wandering Aengus, The," 30, 31, 114
"Sorcerers, The," 86
Speckled Bird, The, 59, 60n3
"Stare's Nest by My Window, The," 66n9, 79–86
"Stirring of the Bones, The," 23n10, 59, 60n3
"Stolen Child, The," 18, 19n3, 31, 73

Yeats, William Butler (*cont.*)
Stories of the Red Hanrahan, The, 108
"Symbolism of Poetry, The," 27
"To be Carved on a Stone at Thoor Ballylee," 53, 62n4, 77, 77n23, 79n26
"To the Rose upon the Rood of Time," 51, 52
"Tower, The" (poem), 58, 58n1
Tower, The (poetry collection), 54, 62n4, 66n9, 83
Trembling of the Veil, The, 23n10, 36, 59, 60n3, 85n40, 189
Uncollected Prose, 58n1, 121
Vision, A, 179
Wanderings of Oisin, The, 8, 18, 19n3, 21, 24–28, 24n11, 24n12, 26n15, 26n16, 31, 32, 38, 39, 41–43, 46, 50–54, 118, 172, 193
Wanderings of Usheen, The, 19n3, 24
Where There is Nothing, 51n37
Wild Swans at Coole, The, 27
Wind Among the Reeds, The, 30, 108
Winding Stair, The, 58n1
Youth, 8, 18, 19, 23n10, 25, 34, 36, 37, 42, 50, 51, 58–59, 60n3, 65–68, 75, 85n40, 106–112, 118–121

The manufacturer's authorised representative in the EU is Springer
Nature Customer Service Centre GmbH, Europaplatz 3, 69115 Heidelberg,
Germany. If you have any concerns regarding our products, please
contact ProductSafety@springernature.com

Printed and bound by CPI Group (UK) Ltd, Croydon, CR0 4YY
01/10/2026
02225953-0004